HEALTH U.

A Nutrition Curriculum for Teenagers with Intellectual Disabilities

Linda Bandini, PhD, RD, Carol Curtin, MSW, Richard Fleming, PhD, Melissa Maslin, MEd, & Renee Scampini, MS, RD

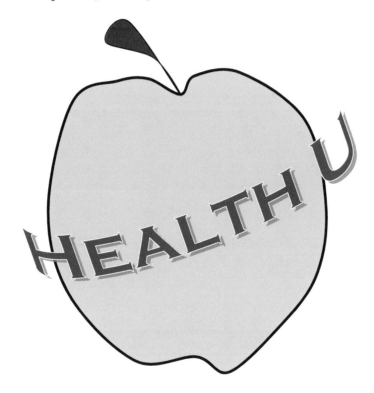

University of Massachusetts Medical School
Eunice Kennedy Shriver Center

ACKNOWLEDGEMENT

We would like to acknowledge and thank former Boston University nutrition graduate students Elizabeth Jordan-Reverri, Lauren Kennedy, Stephanie Parker, and Leslie Song for their contributions to this project.

PROJECT FUNDING

The development of the Health U. curriculum would not have been possible without support from the following organizations: John Alden Trust, National Institute of Diabetes and Digestive and Kidney Diseases, Maternal Child Health Bureau/Leadership Education in Neurodevelopmental Disabilities, Deborah Munroe Noonan Memorial Research Fund, and the Administration on Intellectual and Developmental Disabilities/University Center for Excellence in Developmental Disabilities.

TABLE OF CONTENTS

PREFACE

Purpose of the Health U. Curriculum

Youth with intellectual disabilities (ID) living at home or in the community need to develop the skills necessary to maintain a healthy lifestyle. The first step in developing these skills is to provide individuals with relevant knowledge about eating healthy and the importance of physical activity. Although there is an abundance of nutrition education materials for typically developing adolescents, there is a lack of nutrition education materials geared specifically toward adolescents with ID. Nutrition education programs designed to address this population's cognitive and communicative needs are likely to be more effective than attempts to modify existing curricula.

This curriculum provides age-appropriate nutrition education materials for adolescents and young adults with mild to moderate ID. The curriculum assumes that students will have basic literacy skills (i.e., the ability to read simple words and perform simple measurements). It includes ten lessons, each of which provides a short discussion where new concepts are introduced, an activity that includes hands-on learning, time to engage in movement/physical activity, and a "taste test." The curriculum includes both basic and more advanced activities to accommodate a wide variety of abilities. Instructors can mix and match these activities according to the needs of their students. Finally, there is a "Take Home Ideas" sheet that students fill out at the end of the lesson so they can share what they learned with their parents.

Instructor Qualifications

The curriculum is designed to be taught by registered dietitians or by educators who have had at least two college courses in nutrition. Instructors should have a working knowledge of the USDA's "MyPlate" guidelines, the key nutrients in food groups, and healthy cooking and menu planning skills. It is also recommended that they have some background and experience in working with adolescents or young adults with ID. To help instructors implement the curriculum, we have created a set of guidelines and instructional tips that appear in the lessons themselves.

Curriculum Overview

The curriculum consists of ten 60-minute lessons, which build upon each other and thus should be taught sequentially. Lessons can be delivered on a weekly basis or at intervals appropriate for the group and facility. Each lesson is comprised of 5 sections: Introduction, Activity, Keep Moving, Taste Test, and Daily Wrap-Up. Each section is described briefly below.

> *Introduction*: This section in each lesson provides a very brief (5-10 minutes) presentation in which a new concept is presented. The steps outlined in each introduction section are meant to be a guide; instructors may wish to develop their own interactive discussion-based questions based on the key points listed at the beginning of each introduction. Use of visuals (pictures, flashcards, and food models) throughout the presentation is encouraged to help promote comprehension and sustain students' interest. In later lessons, the introduction section is used to provide a review of previously learned content. Because the activity portions of the lesson are

designed to expand on the students' understanding of the topics introduced here, it is important to keep this introduction brief while making sure that the topics are covered sufficiently.

Activity: Each lesson includes hands-on, interactive activities that meet the lesson objectives. Some lessons have just one activity; others have several shorter activities. Overall, the activity portion is about 30 minutes in duration. Activities are labeled "Level 1" and "Level 2." Level 1 activities are designed for students who have never been exposed to the nutrition concepts presented in the lesson; Level 2 activities are for students who have prior knowledge and/or experience, have mastered the more basic concepts, and are ready for a more advanced activity.

Keep Moving: While the curriculum focuses primarily on nutrition, it also includes an emphasis on the importance of regular physical activity for a healthy lifestyle. Engaging in 15 minutes of simple indoor activities in each lesson stresses the need for being both nutritionally and physically healthy.

Taste Test: Taste tests provide an opportunity for students to try novel foods, especially fruits and vegetables. The taste test for each lesson is thematically related to the lesson topic. After each taste test, students are given an opportunity to rate how they liked the food on a picture scale.

Daily Wrap-Up: Students can share what they learned in class with their parents/caregivers by filling out a "Take Home Ideas" sheet (Appendix E). The sheet has a place for students to write what they learned, what foods they tried in class, and what food they are encouraged to try at home that week.

Note that in some cases, there is more than one introduction and activity in a given lesson. Depending on the time available, instructors may choose to shorten or even eliminate certain parts of the lesson in order to cover topics in sufficient detail or to meet the needs of their students. It is also possible to break longer lessons into two in order to cover all of the parts.

GUIDELINES FOR USE

Instructor Guidelines

The curriculum is structured around simple messages to adopt a healthy lifestyle. These messages may be new to some students, so it is important that the sessions proceed at a pace that will support students' comprehension of the content. The curriculum is designed to be interactive and to promote discussion. A positive, nonjudgmental classroom atmosphere that encourages participation allows students to ask questions and share their experiences and knowledge. Students who have cognitive challenges may need extra time to process information and to formulate responses.

Sessions work best in a small group setting. The lessons contained in this curriculum are geared toward groups of 5 students. For larger groups, more than one instructor may be needed to assist with materials and activities. All lessons include interactive, hands-on activities.

Visual Materials

The use of visual materials promotes comprehension and retention of new information as well as engagement with activities. The interactive lessons are designed to introduce visual and physical representations of food. For example, rather than simply talking about healthy eating and practices such as filling half a plate with fruits and vegetables, students practice this skill by filling half of a real plate with fruit and vegetables. Visuals and manipulatives include pictures, food models, or real food, depending on the instructor's resources. Individuals with ID often have limited literacy skills and benefit from the regular use of visual and hands-on materials to promote their learning. Below are some suggestions for using visual materials in the sessions:

1. Use food models rather than pictures as often as possible. Models are very similar to real food and students are often engaged by just looking at them. To acquire food models:
   a. As your budget allows, order plastic and rubber food models from companies that offer nutrition education materials.
   b. Ask students in the beginning of the program to bring in empty containers of some of their favorite foods and beverages so that they can be incorporated into later lessons.
   c. Supplement plastic food models by saving clean frozen meal boxes, cartons, wrappers and making them as life-like as possible. Examples:
      i. For an empty bag of spinach, fill with green tissue paper so it is shaped and feels like a full bag of spinach.
      ii. For a fast food strawberry smoothie, wrap paper pink paper through the inside of a plastic cup.
      iii. For a microwavable meal, find and cut out pictures of each item in the meal to keep inside the frozen dinner box. Then you can discuss each item individually.
2. There are a number of lessons that require the use of pictures. Included in the appendix are a set of pictures (Appendix C) but instructors may also wish to find additional pictures to tailor specific lessons to their class. Pictures should be clear (not pixilated) and large enough to see from at least five feet away (use the size of Appendix C pictures for reference).

3. Make pictures easy to manipulate:
   a. Laminate pictures so they can be physically maneuvered and handled as opposed to simply viewed.
   b. When pictures need to be posted and moved around for an activity at the front of the classroom, use a cork, magnetic, or felt board and attach the picture with tacks, magnets, or Velcro. This will be easier to see than laying items on a table or passing them around.
4. Be aware of any students who have visual limitations and make accommodations as necessary.
5. For pictures that are to be pasted and glued, some students may enjoy searching for items and cutting them out of magazines, grocery ads, or newspapers.
6. Videos are an excellent way to view how food is prepared, especially for cooking techniques such as deep frying. Search for videos or video clips that are clear without a lot of dialogue.

Shopping

Some lessons may lend themselves to shopping beforehand, though this is not an integral part of the program. If students shop for groceries, make a smaller version of vocabulary word flashcards (Appendix A) that students can reference while shopping. Laminate and clip together with a ring so students can easily flip through the words at the store.

Classroom Set-Up

In each lesson, the Materials and Preparation section provides very specific materials needed and classroom set-up. The set-up for Keep Moving, Taste Test, and Daily Wrap-Up sections are standard in each lesson and are described below.

Keep Moving

Physical activity is as important to health as nutrition. Using 15 minutes during each class to engage in a brief physical activity provides students with ideas for easy physical activities to try at home and reinforces the importance of physical activity. Appendix F has a list of physical activities that can be done in the classroom with little to no set-up time or equipment.

The Keep Moving portion of the class occurs after the nutrition part of the lesson is over. Instructors can propose one or two physical activity ideas, and either take a vote, or ask one student each week to decide what the activity will be. After a few weeks of class, these ideas can be used as springboards to brainstorm other ideas. Dancing is popular and easy; instructors can encourage students to bring in their favorite music. Instructors can lead by example and join the activity, reinforce the importance of doing physical activities at home, and encourage students to stay moving even if they are getting tired.

Taste Tests

All lessons include "taste tests" to provide an opportunity for students to make and sample healthy foods, especially fruits and vegetables. After the taste test, students will have an opportunity to rate the food on the "Take Home Ideas" sheet that is sent home after each session (see Appendix E).

Below are some suggestions for implementing the taste tests:

1. **_CHECK FOR ALLERGIES_** and/or dietary restrictions before offering any food.
2. Remain culturally sensitive by incorporating foods that students and their families eat.
3. Be aware of and accommodate any chewing or swallowing problems that students may have.
4. Choose foods that students are familiar with, as well as a few the instructor believes they may have never seen before. The goal is to help expand students' food repertoires. Students who are reluctant to try a novel food may be willing to try something familiar, so a combination of new and familiar foods is recommended. Also, seeing foods in a different environment with peers who can provide encouragement may make students more willing to try new foods.
5. Present foods in a fun and attractive way, such as using colorful napkins or a swirly, tropical straw for smoothie drinks.
6. Recipes that accompany the taste tests have few steps and ingredients and can be followed by students with minimal supervision. Instructors can send home copies of the recipes with the students.
7. For class periods longer than an hour, involve students in the preparation of the taste test.

Daily Wrap-Up

This is an opportunity for the instructor to review what was learned in class, as well as for students to complete a "Take Home Ideas" sheet (Appendix E) to bring home. Students will fill in with words or pictures what they learned that day, what food(s) they tried, and how they liked it. The sheet also suggests a food for the teen to try at home so parents/caregivers can continue to support the teen in trying new healthy foods. Like the taste test, the food is thematically tied to the lesson. For example, after learning about fruits and vegetables, students are encouraged to try a new vegetable at home that week.

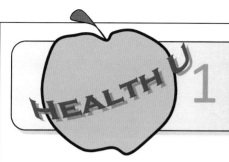

HEALTH 1 — Introduction to Nutrition and MyPlate

OVERVIEW

The goal of this lesson is to get students thinking about why nutrition is important for them. It lays the groundwork for future lessons. This class introduces new nutrition terms, the five food groups, and the "MyPlate" model.

LEARNING OBJECTIVES

At the end of the session, students will be able to:
- ✓ Describe the meaning of the terms nutrition, energy, variety, and vitamins
- ✓ Identify the five food groups and name some foods in each group
- ✓ Identify the components of MyPlate
- ✓ Explain the importance of good nutrition

MATERIALS AND PREPARATION

General Materials for Lesson

Appendix Materials
- Flashcards with each of the following terms on one side, and the definition on the other: nutrition, energy, vitamins, and variety (Appendix A)
- 5 food group cards (Appendix B)
- Printed photographs of individual foods from all five food groups (Appendix C)
- Image of MyPlate (Appendix D)
- "Take Home Ideas" worksheet (Appendix E)
- Physical activity ideas (Appendix F)

Additional Materials (see Guidelines for Use, p. iii, for tips on obtaining these)
- Additional images of food items from each food group
- Plastic food models and/or real food boxes/containers from each food group
- Large (at least 27" x 39") poster or representation of MyPlate

1. Introduction to Nutrition and MyPlate

MATERIALS AND PREPARATION

Activity-Specific Materials and Preparation

Activity 1.2

Materials

Appendix Materials
- 5 food group cards (Appendix B)

Additional Materials
- Plastic food models and real foods/food containers for foods from all 5 groups, enough for each student to participate a few times
  - *Note: If real foods and food containers and/or plastic food models are not available, you can use pictures from Appendix C as well as ones you've acquired.*
- A large box with a lid
- 5 empty bins (clean garbage cans, additional boxes)

Preparation
1. Cut a 6x6" hole in the lid of the box.
2. Fill the box with a variety of food models from all five food groups. Place the lid on top.
3. Label the five empty bins with the five food group cards so the items can be sorted into the appropriate food groups.

Activity 1.3A

Materials

Appendix Materials
- Printed MyPlate, one for each student (Appendix D)

Additional Materials
- Small cut-out pictures of food items from each food group
- White paper plates and cups that are close to the size of MyPlate print-out, one for each student
- Glue sticks and tape

Preparation
1. Cut out each section of the MyPlate (protein, grain, vegetable, fruit, dairy) for each student before class.
2. Sort food pictures into food groups.

1.   Introduction to Nutrition and MyPlate

MATERIALS AND PREPARATION

Activity 1.3B
Materials
Appendix Materials
- 5 food group cards (Appendix B)

Additional Materials
- One lunch bag per student
- Food models or pictures of items to make up a lunch (examples below)

Preparation
1. Fill at least one bag per student with food from only 4 different food groups.
   EXAMPLES of brown bag lunches with a missing food group:
   - Grain missing: Pear, carrot sticks, yogurt, nuts
   - Fruit missing: Veggie soup, cheese stick, crackers, hardboiled egg
   - Vegetable missing: Banana, ham and cheese sandwich
   - Protein missing: Applesauce, milk, roll, small salad
   - Dairy missing: Raisins, salsa, tortilla chips, black beans
2. Have additional food pictures and models at the front of the room to "complete" the meal.
3. Tips for creating lunches:
   - Keep lunches realistic by choosing items that students might bring in a bag lunch.
   - Be culturally sensitive: choose foods based on your location and the racial-ethnic composition of your class to ensure students will recognize the foods in the lunches.
   - Avoid combination foods (e.g., pizza), as they are covered in later lessons and may cause confusion. Sandwiches may be appropriate if each of the pieces can be pulled apart and identified.

SECTION 1.1: INTRODUCTION TO HEALTHY EATING

This section focuses on the importance of good nutrition. Lead a short (5-10 minute) discussion on the impact of healthy eating on the students' lives. The purpose of this exercise is to start an open dialogue about nutrition and what it means to eat healthy.

Key Points:
- Nutrition is the science of healthy food choices, and learning about it helps us make these choices.
- Healthy foods give us energy to fuel our bodies and vitamins to keep us healthy.
- We know we're eating in a healthy way when we choose foods with the right balance of energy and vitamins.

1. Start by asking the students, "What does the word **nutrition** mean to you?" (hold up corresponding flashcard).
2. Explain that nutrition is the science of healthy food choices, and learning about nutrition helps us make these choices.
3. Ask the students to explain why we need to eat food. Use the analogy of putting gas in a car to illustrate the concept of energy.
4. Ask the students if they know why we should eat healthy foods.
5. Explain that healthy foods give us **energy** (hold up flashcard) to fuel our bodies and **vitamins** (hold up flashcard) to keep us healthy.
6. Ask students how we know we're eating healthy foods.
7. Explain that we know we're eating in a healthy way when we choose foods with the right balance of energy and vitamins.

LESSON TIPS

✓ Wait/prompt for student comments and answers (this may take time).

✓ Use food pictures and models for students to reference.

SECTION 1.2: DISCUSSION OF THE FIVE FOOD GROUPS

This section introduces the five food groups, covered in much more detail later. For now, students should only be able to name all five groups and, by the end of this lesson, to categorize foods into the correct group.

1. Explain to the students that foods can be separated into five different food groups, and today they are going to learn about each one of them.
2. Start with the fruits group. Hold up the large **fruits** card, and ask students if they can name any foods that belong in that group. If students have a hard time coming up with examples, name a couple.
3. Next, hold up the large **vegetables** card, and ask students if they can name any vegetables. Again, if they have trouble thinking of examples, provide some of your own.
4. Move on to the **dairy** card and follow the same procedure.
5. Next, hold up the **grains** card and ask students for examples, etc.
6. Finally, show the students the **protein** card. Explain that this is sometimes called the meat or the meat and beans group. Ask them for examples and provide some of your own.

LESSON TIP

✓ If the students in your class find the pictures to be too visually overwhelming, you may wish to use food models or individual pictures of foods that can be found in Appendix C.

At this point in the lesson, transition into the activity.

ACTIVITY 1.2: LEVEL 1, KNOWLEDGE-CENTERED ACTIVITY

In this activity, students will participate in a hands-on activity to identify and categorize foods into the five food groups. The activity is designed to engage the students by having surprises and challenges. Students reach in to a covered box that is filled with food models, and they can only feel the food – they can't see it. Each student should have the chance to pick a food out of the box, identify it, and place it in the correct bin. Students will eventually identify more challenging foods, such as combination foods, which fall into more than one food group.

1. One student at a time chooses a food model out of the box and identifies it.
2. The student then names the food group that the food belongs to and places it in the correct bin. He or she can ask classmates for help if unsure.
3. Correct wrong answers.
4. Repeat until all of the students have participated at least a few times.

REMEMBER

✓ Level 1 activities are designed for students who have never been exposed to nutrition concepts.

✓ Level 2 activities are designed for students who have mastered the concept of categorizing food into food groups.

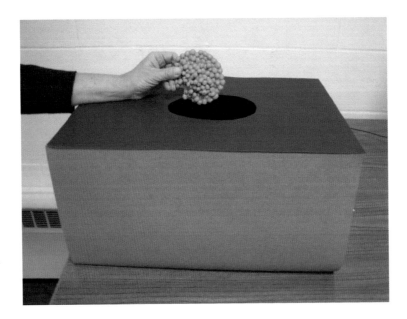

SECTION 1.3: INTRODUCTION TO MYPLATE

This section introduces MyPlate (Appendix D) from the ChooseMyPlate.gov website as a model for healthy eating and variety. Emphasize that this tool is a guide for fixing a plate at a meal. For this lesson, teach only what each space on the plate represents. Students are taught later how to use the MyPlate as a model for selecting foods and appropriate portion sizes at meals.

Key Points:
- MyPlate can help us choose foods that will make a healthy meal because it includes all of the food groups.
- We need to eat these different foods because they each have different vitamins. By eating foods from all food groups, we can get all the vitamins we need to be healthy. This is called variety, which means eating foods from all food groups every day for good health.

1. Show students the MyPlate poster and explain that it can be used as a model to help us choose foods that will make a healthy meal.
2. Point out each part of the MyPlate and explain what it represents. For example, "This plate has all the food groups on it. Let's look at the colors to see what they represent. The green part of the plate is for vegetables and the red part is for fruits. Notice how these food groups take up half the plate. The orange part is for grains. The purple part is for protein foods. These two groups take up the other half of your plate. Dairy is on the side because we usually have dairy by drinking milk or eating yogurt."
3. Give an example of a MyPlate with all five food groups represented. Ask the students if they can think of another example of a meal with all five groups.
4. Ask the students why it might be important to have all of the food groups in one meal.
5. Explain that we need to eat these different foods because they each have different vitamins (hold up flashcard). By eating foods from all food groups, we can get all the vitamins we need to be healthy. This is called **variety** (hold up flashcard), which means eating foods from all food groups every day for good health.

LESSON TIPS

✓Encourage participation by engaging all the students in the discussion and activity.

✓Use a large MyPlate.gov poster and food pictures for students to reference. Put food pictures in the corresponding color section of the plate.

ACTIVITY 1.3A: LEVEL 1, KNOWLEDGE-CENTERED ACTIVITY

This activity will provide students with their own healthy plate model.

1. Students attach the orange, purple, and green sections of MyPlate to their paper plate, and the blue section to the cup.
2. Ask the students to choose a food that they like from each food group and attach a picture of it to the corresponding section on their plate, one in each section.
3. Throughout the activity, review how this model can help them choose their meals and make sure they get enough variety.

Note: If having the students glue the sections of MyPlate onto their plates and cups will be too time consuming, prepare plates before class, and have students only attach food pictures.

> **REMEMBER**
>
> ✓ Level 1 activities are designed for students who have never been exposed to nutrition concepts.
>
> ✓ Level 2 activities are designed for students who have mastered the concept of categorizing food into food groups.

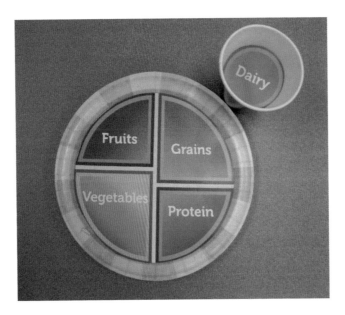

ACTIVITY 1.3B: LEVEL 2, KNOWLEDGE-CENTERED ACTIVITY

In this "brown bag lunch" game, students will search through pre-made bag lunches containing 4 items, each from a specific food group. One food group is missing from the bag, so the student must identify the missing one. This activity will help students practice their food categorizing skills and reinforces the concept of variety.

1. One at a time, each student empties a bag lunch and determines which food group is missing.
2. Encourage the student to use the 5 food group cards to identify which food groups are already in the lunch, which will help him or her find the missing one.
3. Once the student knows which food group is missing, he or she completes the meal by choosing a food from the missing group.
4. Repeat until each student has had a turn.

REMEMBER

✓ Level 1 activities are designed for students who have never been exposed to nutrition concepts.

✓ Level 2 activities are designed for students who have mastered the concept of categorizing food into food groups.

"KEEP MOVING"

Take 15 minutes at the end of class to participate in an interactive physical activity (see Appendix F for ideas).

PHYSICAL ACTIVITY TIP

Give a pep talk about how physical activity goes hand-in-hand with good nutrition for health. Explain that physical activity can be very fun and should be done daily.

If resources are available, try to conclude each lesson with a taste test. Taste test ideas:

- **Vegetables or fruits that are in season**
- **Sampler of (small) servings from each of the five food groups**

TASTE TEST TIP

Encourage students to *try* new foods by explaining that they don't need to like the food, they only have to try it. It can take dozens of tries to acquire a taste for a given food, so it is helpful to repeat exposures to new foods. Keep this in mind when selecting foods for the "taste test" at the conclusion of each lesson.

DAILY WRAP-UP (Appendix E)

Try a new food from one of the food groups!

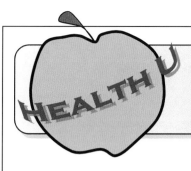

2 Fruits, Vegetables, and Dairy

OVERVIEW

This lesson highlights three food groups: fruits, vegetables, and dairy, as part of a healthy diet. For fruits and vegetables, the main focus is on variety and eating fruits and vegetables from all colors of the rainbow. For dairy, the main focus is on eating dairy often (at every meal). This lesson also allows students to practice the skill(s) of either grocery shopping through an online vendor and/or finding vegetables on a restaurant menu.

LEARNING OBJECTIVES

At the end of the session, students will be able to:
- ✓ Identify foods in the fruit, vegetable, and dairy groups
- ✓ Explain the importance of eating fruits, vegetables, and dairy
- ✓ Use a shopping list to find items at an online grocer and/or find vegetables on a restaurant menu

MATERIALS AND PREPARATION

General Materials for Lesson
Appendix Materials
- Flashcard with each of the following terms on one side and the definition on the other: vitamins, variety (Appendix A)
- Fruits, Vegetables, and Dairy food group cards (Appendix B)
- Printed photographs of individual foods from all three food groups (Appendix C)
- Image of MyPlate (Appendix D)
- "Take Home Ideas" worksheet (Appendix E)
- Physical activity ideas (Appendix F)

Additional Materials (see Guidelines for Use, p. iii, for tips on obtaining these)
- Additional images of fruits, vegetables, and dairy foods
- Plastic food models, real foods, or real food containers (fresh and frozen fruits and vegetables, dairy and non-dairy – soy, almond, or rice-based – milk and yogurt)

2. Fruits, Vegetables, and Dairy

MATERIALS AND PREPARATION

Activity-Specific Materials and Preparation

Activity 2.1A
Materials
Appendix Materials
- "Eat a Rainbow" placemat template (Appendix G), one for each student
- Small pictures of different-colored fruits and vegetables, enough for each student to choose three or four (Appendix C)

Additional Materials
- Additional small pictures of fruits and vegetables
- Glue sticks
- 7 small bowls for sorting pictures of fruits and vegetables

Preparation
1. Separate the fruit and vegetable pictures by color (red, orange, yellow, green, blue, purple, white) and place them in separate bowls.

Activity 2.1B
Materials (choose one)
Appendix Materials
- Sample food menu (Appendix H)

Additional Materials
- Actual food menu from a local restaurant, one copy for each student

Activity 2.2A
Materials
Appendix Materials – None
Additional Materials
- Computer with internet access
- Projector (optional)
- Any adaptive materials available (depending on the needs of the students)

Preparation
1. Create a shopping list with at least one fruit or vegetable that is fresh, canned, and frozen, and 3 dairy items.
   > Sample grocery list: tomatoes, bananas, applesauce, frozen broccoli, canned green beans, skim milk, yogurt, cheddar cheese
2. Find an online grocer at www.mywebgrocer.com and familiarize yourself with the grocer ahead of time.

SECTION 2.1: FRUITS AND VEGETABLES

This section focuses on fruits and vegetables and why we should eat a variety of different colors of fruits and vegetables daily, an idea that is captured by the phrase "Eat a rainbow every day!", an easy reminder to eat different-colored fruits and vegetables.

Key Messages:

- We should fill half our plate with fruits and vegetables.
- Fruits and vegetables help us feel full longer so that we're less hungry between meals and snacks. They have lots of vitamins and minerals, which keep our bodies healthy and help fight off colds and other infections.
- It's important to eat a variety of fruits and vegetables, in all different colors, every day, so that we can get all of the vitamins we need. Remember to "Eat a rainbow every day!"

Sample discussion:

1. Remind the students of MyPlate and explain that today we're going to focus on the fruits and vegetables section of MyPlate. Ask them how much of our plate we should fill with fruits and vegetables.
2. Ask students *why* they think we should fill half our plates with fruits and vegetables; in other words, why do we need to eat so many fruits and vegetables every day?
3. Explain that fruits and vegetables help us feel full longer so that we're less hungry between meals and snacks. They also have lots of **vitamins** (hold up flashcard) and minerals, which keep our bodies healthy and help fight off colds and other infections.
4. Explain that it's really important to eat a **variety** (hold up flashcard) of fruits and vegetables every day, because different colored fruits and vegetables give us different vitamins. For example, orange vegetables are good for our eyes, and red fruits help fight off colds. So we need to eat all the different colors of fruits and vegetables so that we can get all of the vitamins we need to stay healthy.
5. Tell the students that one good way to remember to eat a variety of colors is to remember to "eat a rainbow every day!", which means that we should remember to eat fruits and vegetables of all colors of the rainbow.
6. Ask students to name the colors of a rainbow, making sure that all of them are listed.
7. Now ask the students to think about different fruits and vegetables, and to name some red ones. Repeat with orange, yellow, green, blue, purple, and white.

LESSON TIPS

- ✓ Wait and prompt for student comments and answers.
- ✓ Use food pictures and models for students to reference.

At this point in the lesson, transition into the activity.

ACTIVITY 2.1A: LEVEL 1, KNOWLEDGE-CENTERED ACTIVITY

This activity will help reinforce the importance of eating a variety of different-colored fruits and vegetables every day.

1. Ask students to select at least one fruit or vegetable from each bowl (one bowl per color).
2. Students should then glue the fruit(s)/vegetable(s) they've selected onto their placemats, so that they make a rainbow on their plates.
3. Monitor each student's progress to make sure he or she has selected a fruit/vegetable for each color (red, orange, yellow, green, blue, purple, and white). If one or more color is missing, prompt student to identify it and find a fruit or vegetable to represent it.
4. Ask students to show their placemats to each other and describe what they put on their plates.

REMEMBER

✓ Level 1 activities are designed for students who have never been exposed to nutrition concepts.

✓ Level 2 activities are designed for students who have mastered the concept of categorizing food into food groups.

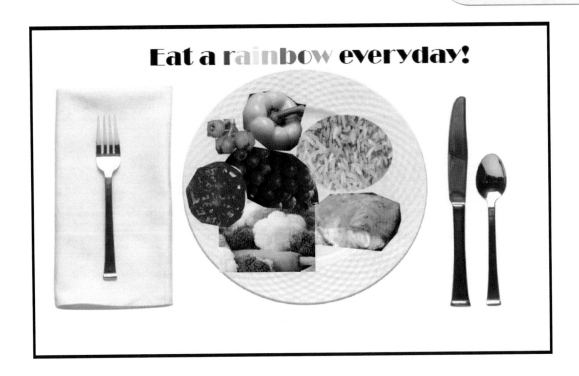

ACTIVITY 2.1B: LEVEL 2, SKILL-CENTERED ACTIVITY

In this activity, students will practice finding healthy items on a restaurant menu.

1. Distribute a copy of a restaurant menu to each student.
2. Ask the students to find all of the dishes with vegetables in them.
3. For meals without a vegetable, ask the students how they could substitute a vegetable for another item (e.g., getting green beans instead of French fries) or add a vegetable (e.g., a side salad) to add variety to the meal.

ACTIVITY TIPS

✓ A sample menu is provided in Appendix H, but it is best to use a local restaurant with which students are familiar.

✓ Choose menus that use simple language and are not visually complex.

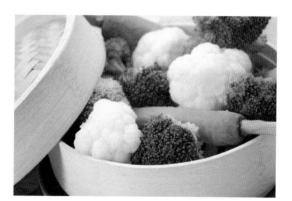

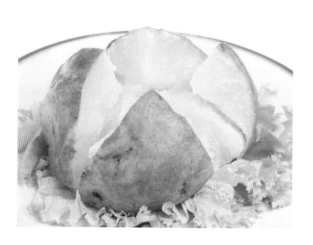

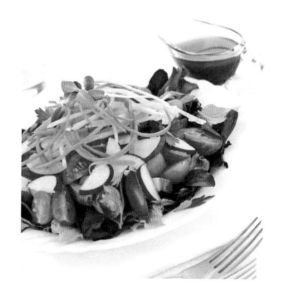

SECTION 2.2: DAIRY

This section focuses on the importance of dairy, identifying dairy foods and the number of times (3) we should consume dairy each day.

Key Points:
- We should drink milk or eat dairy three times a day.
- Milk and other dairy items have calcium and vitamin D, which help build strong bones and teeth.

1. Ask students to name some foods that are in the dairy group.
2. Ask, "Does anyone know how many times a day we should drink milk or eat dairy?" If no one provides the correct answer, tell the students that we should drink milk or eat dairy three times a day, and explain that a good way to remember this is to eat dairy with every meal.
3. Ask whether anyone knows how drinking milk helps our bodies; in other words, why is it important to drink milk or eat dairy three times a day?
4. Explain that milk and other dairy items have calcium and vitamin D, which help build strong bones and teeth.

L E S S O N   T I P S

✓ Wait/prompt for student comments and answers (this may take time).

✓ Use the Dairy food group card and/or food models and pictures as visual examples.

✓ If any of your students do not eat dairy for medical or other reasons (e.g., lactose intolerance, a casein-free or vegan diet, etc.), discuss fortified almond or soy milk as possible alternatives to dairy.

ACTIVITY 2.2A: LEVEL 2, SKILL-CENTERED ACTIVITY

Students will practice locating fruits, vegetables, and dairy while grocery shopping online.

1. Log on to online grocer.
2. Using a shopping list, ask students to find the items listed and add them to the online shopping cart.
3. Encourage student interaction and tailor the activity to their abilities and the resources of the classroom. For example, students may be able to take turns clicking on grocery items and adding them to a basket, or you can actually add the foods to the cart while asking students which "aisles" might have the foods on the shopping list.

ACTIVITY TIP

✓ Students may not know some vocabulary words (for example, "produce"), so be prepared to define terminology that is website-specific.

2. Fruits, Vegetables, and Dairy

"KEEP MOVING"

Take 15 minutes at the end of class to participate in an interactive physical activity (see Appendix F for ideas).

PHYSICAL ACTIVITY TIP
Play dance music to encourage movement.

If resources are available, try to conclude each lesson with a taste test. Taste test ideas:

Smoothies with yogurt and frozen fruit
Recipe:
1 part milk, 1 part plain yogurt
2 parts frozen fruit or fresh fruit and ice

Non-dairy alternatives can be used if students are lactose intolerant but do not have soy or nut allergies.

TASTE TEST TIP
These are a favorite, be sure to have enough!

DAILY WRAP-UP (Appendix E)

Try a new vegetable at lunch or dinner!

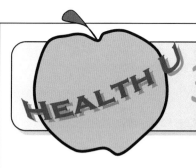

Grains and Protein

3

OVERVIEW

The goal of this lesson is to explore grains and protein; the priority here is to teach students how to identify the wide variety of foods that fall into each of these categories. Whole grains are introduced in this lesson as a healthier choice than refined grains, but lean sources of protein are introduced in later lessons (6 and 7).

LEARNING OBJECTIVES

At the end of the session, students will be able to:
- ✓ Identify whole grains and refined grains
- ✓ Explain why whole grains are the healthiest choice
- ✓ Categorize foods into the protein (meat and beans) group
- ✓ Explain why we need to eat grains and protein

MATERIALS AND PREPARATION

General Materials for the Lesson
Appendix Materials
- Flashcards with each of the following terms on one side and the definition on the other: energy, vitamins, fiber, whole grains, white grains (Appendix A)
- Protein and Grains food group cards (Appendix B)
- Printed photographs of individual foods from the protein and grains groups (Appendix C)
- Image of MyPlate (Appendix D)
- Whole grain model (Appendix I)
- "Take Home Ideas" worksheet (Appendix E)
- Physical activity ideas (Appendix F)

Additional Materials (see Guidelines for Use, p. iii, for tips on obtaining these)
- Additional images of proteins (examples of each type: meat, fish, beans, nuts, and eggs) and grains (as many different types as possible)
- Plastic food models and real foods or food containers of proteins and grains, including: slices of white and wheat bread, empty tuna and bean cans, egg carton, peanut butter jar, boxes of rice and pasta

3. Grains and Protein

MATERIALS AND PREPARATION

Activity-Specific Materials and Preparation

Activity 3.1A

Materials

Appendix Materials

- Flashcards with each of the following terms on one side and the definition on the other: whole grains and 100% whole wheat (Appendix A)

Additional Materials

- Plastic food models and real foods or food containers of the following pairs: bags of whole wheat and white bread, packages of brown and white rice, boxes of oatmeal and grits, boxes of whole wheat and white pasta, boxes of corn flakes and shredded wheat, pretzels and popcorn (this one is tricky!)
  - *Note: If real and plastic food models are not available, you can use pictures.*

Activity 3.1B

Materials

Appendix Materials – None

Additional Materials

- Bag of un-popped popcorn kernels
- Microwave
- Small brown paper lunch bags, one for each student
- 1 tablespoon measuring spoon
- Optional: non-stick cooking spray, flavorings (e.g., salt, parmesan cheese, cinnamon and sugar, etc.)

Activity 3.2

Materials

Appendix Materials

- BINGO board, one for each student (Appendix J)
- 5 letter cards labeled with the letter B, I, N, G, or O (Appendix J)
- 5 protein category cards labeled beans, nuts, fish, eggs, or meat, with corresponding pictures (Appendix J)

Additional Materials

- BINGO markers, such as a penny or dried bean (at least 20 per student)

SECTION 3.1: THE GRAINS GROUP

This section highlights 1) why we need grains as part of a healthy diet, 2) the wide variety of grains (from rice to cereal to crackers), and 3) that whole grains are the healthier choice. Focus primarily on how to identify a whole grain.

Key Points:

- Grains give us lots of energy, vitamins, and fiber.
- Whole grains, including whole wheat bread, are healthier than white grains, because they give us more vitamins and fiber.
- To figure out whether you're eating a whole grain instead of a white grain, look for: darker color (whole grains are usually darker than white ones) or the words "whole grain" or "100% whole wheat" on the label.

1. Remind the students of MyPlate and explain that today we're going to focus on the Grains section of MyPlate. Hold up the Grains card and ask the students to name some foods that are in the grains group.
2. Make sure that students are naming a wide variety of grains, and supplement their answers with more diverse examples if they aren't. Explain that there are many different kinds of grains, and they all look pretty different.
3. Ask students why we eat grains. Explain that grains give us lots of **energy** (hold up flashcard) so we can study, work, play, and learn. They also have **vitamins** (hold up flashcard) that are different than the vitamins in other food groups. Grains also have **fiber** (hold up flashcard), which helps our digestive system by keeping our intestines healthy.
4. Hold up two slices of bread, one whole wheat and one white. Ask the students whether they know what kind of bread each one is (to gauge if they are familiar with the terms "whole wheat" and "white"), and if they do, ask if they know what the difference is between them.
5. Ask the students, "Which slice of bread is healthier? Why?"
6. Explain that the whole wheat bread is healthier because it has a lot more vitamins and fiber than white bread. When companies make white bread (or white rice, pasta, crackers), they take away a lot of the vitamins and fiber.
7. Hold up the model of a whole grain (Appendix I), and show students that a whole grain has three parts: the endosperm, which gives us energy; the bran, which gives us fiber; and the germ, which gives us vitamins. **Whole grains** (hold up flashcard), including whole wheat bread, have all three parts, but **white grains** (hold up flashcard) only have the endosperm, so it has almost no fiber or vitamins.
8. Ask students if they know how we can find whole grain foods. Explain that whole grain foods are usually darker than white grain foods, and that they can look for the words "whole grain" or "100% whole wheat" on the food label.

LESSON TIP: ✓ Use food models and images to identify grain items. Be sure to cover a variety of grains because many of them look different: rice, pasta, tortilla, popcorn, oatmeal, bread, crackers etc.

At this point in the lesson, transition into the activity.

ACTIVITY 3.1A: LEVEL 1, KNOWLEDGE-CENTERED ACTIVITY

In this activity, students will be presented with two different grains and asked to find the whole grain.

1. Set up the whole/white grain pairs out on a table.
2. Have one student at a time select a pair of grains from the table.
3. Ask the student, "Which is the whole grain?" of the pair, and why they think that.
4. Correct any wrong answers.
5. Repeat with all pairs of grains.

ACTIVITY TIPS

✓ Make sure the whole grain items look obviously brown for easy identification.

✓ Use flashcards to help the students find words on packaging.

ACTIVITY 3.1B: LEVEL 1, SKILL-CENTERED ACTIVITY

Students will practice cooking popcorn.

1. Explain to students that popcorn is a great healthy, whole grain snack.
2. Give each student an empty lunch bag.
3. Have one student at a time measure 1 tablespoon of popcorn kernels and pour them into the bag.
4. After the kernels are measured, fold the top of the bag 3 times and microwave it using the popcorn setting (or for 1-3 minutes), listening for the popping to slow to a few pops per second.

ACTIVITY TIPS

✓ Usually the popping takes about 2 minutes, but the time can vary depending on the microwave. You may want to try this activity ahead of time so you will know how long it takes to cook popcorn in the microwave you will be using.

✓ Be aware of hot popcorn bags and ask students to handle them with care.

✓ If you decide to flavor the popcorn, coat the popped kernels with cooking spray and then shake the flavoring into the bag after it has been popped. Invite the students to try a little bit of each flavor.

✓ This activity provides an opportunity to review food safety practices such as hand washing.

SECTION 3.2: THE PROTEIN GROUP

This section highlights why protein is important and which foods are in the protein group. Make sure to cover all foods that are sources of protein: meat, fish, legumes, nuts, and eggs.

Key Points:
- Protein helps us stay healthy and strong by building our organs, tissues, and muscles.
- There are many different kinds of protein foods – not just meat and beans.

1. Show the students the Protein section of MyPlate. Ask them, "When I say the word 'protein,' what foods do you think of?"
2. If the students focus mainly on meat, or meat and beans, explain that there are many different kinds of protein foods. Sometimes the protein food group is called the "meat and beans" group, but there's even more than just meat and beans in it. Show them the protein food group card and ask them to try to name all the different kinds of protein they can.
3. Explain that protein helps us stay healthy and strong by building our organs, tissues, and muscles. The foods in the protein group all look, taste, and feel pretty different, so it's important to learn which foods are part of the protein group.

LESSON TIPS

✓ Wait/prompt for student comments and answers (this may take time).

✓ Rely heavily on food models and images, as protein foods are very tricky to categorize due to their great variety.

✓ Help students build on their answers in order to identify all the types of protein.

ACTIVITY 3.2A: LEVEL 1, KNOWLEDGE-CENTERED ACTIVITY

Students will play BINGO with the large variety of protein foods.

1. Pass out BINGO boards and markers to the students and have them cover the middle "free protein" square with a marker.
2. Explain the BINGO rules.
3. Randomly select a letter card and a category card and call out the combination (e.g., "N, beans"). As you call the category, hold up pictures of examples of those proteins as a visual reminder. If a student has that type of protein in that letter column (e.g., has a picture of pinto beans in the column under the letter "N"), they should mark their board. Keep track of each combination to reference later.
4. Continue step #2 until someone calls "BINGO!" – five marked spaces in a row either vertically, horizontally, or diagonally. Ask the student to share what they marked under each combination you called (e.g., ask what food they marked under "N" for beans) to further review what foods are in the protein group. You may need to assist students with labeling the individual foods (e.g., pinto beans).
5. Continue until everyone has had BINGO at least once.

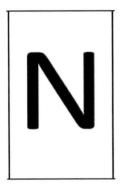

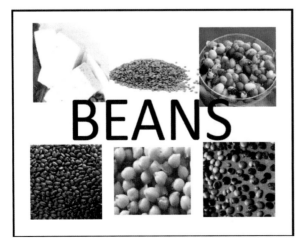

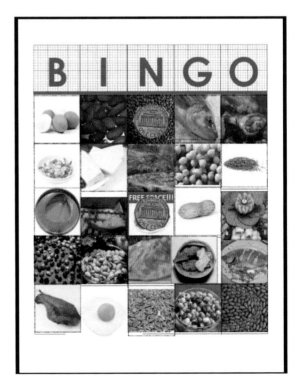

"KEEP MOVING"

Take 15 minutes at the end of class to participate in an interactive physical activity (see Appendix F for ideas).

PHYSICAL ACTIVITY TIP
Encourage students to do their favorite physical activities at home.

If resources are available, try to conclude each lesson with a taste test. Taste test ideas:

· Popcorn!
· Whole grain sampler (quinoa, bulgar, brown rice, whole wheat pasta); whole grain crackers with tuna or shrimp salad; hummus and veggies or pita chips; frozen, flavored tofu such as Tofettes

TASTE TEST TIP
Quinoa and bulgar can be eaten hot or cold and are easy to prepare in advance.

DAILY WRAP-UP (Appendix E)

Eat a new protein food and report how it tastes!

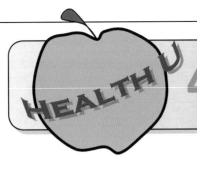

4 Meal Planning: Focus on Variety and Mixed Dishes

OVERVIEW

This lesson builds on the first three lessons. At this point, students should be able to categorize foods in the five food groups. The goal of this lesson is to expand on the students' understanding of the concept of variety among food groups and for them to learn about "mixed dishes" that contain more than one food group. Some common mixed dishes (e.g., pizza, macaroni and cheese) are highlighted and modified as a way to increase variety at a meal.

LEARNING OBJECTIVES

At the end of the session, students will be able to:
- ✓ Explain the concept of variety among food groups
- ✓ Identify the foods in mixed dishes and which food group each belongs to
- ✓ Explain how to increase variety in meals by modifying mixed dishes
- ✓ Plan a menu and grocery list

MATERIALS AND PREPARATION

General Materials for the Lesson

Appendix Materials
- Flashcards with each of the following terms on one side, and the definition on the other: variety, vitamins (Appendix A)
- 5 food group cards (Appendix B)
- Printed photographs of individual foods representing all five food groups (Appendix C)
- Images of 3 different plates with 1, 2, or 3 foods (Appendix K)
- Mixed food examples – cut out, laminated, and assembled (Appendix L)
- "Take Home Ideas" worksheet (Appendix E)
- Physical activity ideas (Appendix F)

Additional Materials (see Guidelines for Use, p. iii, for tips on obtaining these)
- Plastic food models, real boxes of frozen dinners and other mixed dishes
- 3 different plates set up as display meals using food models (if not using Appendix K materials)
  - Meal 1: chicken
  - Meal 2: chicken and rice
  - Meal 3: chicken, rice, and vegetables
- Chalk board and chalk, or white board with markers

4. Meal Planning: Variety and Mixed Dishes

MATERIALS AND PREPARATION

Activity-Specific Materials and Preparation

Activity 4.1A

Materials

Appendix Materials

- 5 food group cards (Appendix B)

Additional Materials

- One brown lunch bag per student
- Food models or pictures of items to make a lunch

Preparation

1. Fill at least one bag per student with food from only 4 different food groups.

    Level 1 Examples:

    > Grain missing: pear, carrot sticks, yogurt, nuts
    >
    > Fruit missing: veggie soup, cheese stick, crackers, hardboiled egg
    >
    > Vegetable missing: banana, ham and cheese sandwich
    >
    > Protein missing: apple sauce, milk, roll, small salad
    >
    > Dairy missing: raisins, salsa, tortilla chips, black beans

    Level 2 Examples: remove 2 or more food groups

2. Tips for creating lunches:
    - Keep lunches realistic by choosing items that students might eat in a bagged lunch.
    - Stay culturally sensitive: choose foods based on your location and the racial-ethnic composition of the class to ensure students will recognize the foods in their brown bag lunches.
    - Avoid combination foods (e.g., pizza) as they are covered in later lessons and may cause confusion. Sandwiches may be appropriate if each one of the pieces can be pulled apart and identified.

3. Have additional food pictures and models at the front of the room to "complete" the meal.

4. Meal Planning: Variety and Mixed Dishes

MATERIALS AND PREPARATION

Activity 4.2A
Materials
Appendix Materials
- 5 food group cards (Appendix B)
- Mixed dish examples, cut out, laminated, and stuck together with tape or Velcro (Appendix L)
- Printed photographs of individual foods representing all five food groups (Appendix C)

Additional Materials
- Additional mixed dishes to categorize
- Additional images of food items to add to the meal
- Dry erase board with markers

Preparation
1. Divide the board into 5 columns, one for each food group. Label columns with the 5 food group cards.
2. Have mixed dishes ready to present to students, and place additional food pictures to complete the meal on an easily-accessible separate table.
    Examples of mixed dishes (Appendix L), in order of increasing difficulty:
    Sandwich: Missing fruit
    Macaroni and cheese: Missing protein, vegetables, and fruit
    Macaroni and red sauce: Missing protein, fruit, and dairy
    Pizza: Missing protein and needs more vegetables
3. Tips for this activity:
    - Develop your own materials based on the dietary habits of the students (e.g., use frozen dinner boxes if they are popular and make individual cut-outs of each part of the dinner).
    - Use real foods that students may eat together, or would go well with the mixed dish (e.g., add a side salad to pizza).
    - Using a magnetic board makes it easy to categorize the mixed dish parts into the correct columns.

Activity 4.2B
Materials
Appendix Materials
- 5 food group cards (Appendix B)
- Printed photographs of individual foods representing all five food groups (Appendix C)

Additional Materials
- Additional images of food items
- Chalk board and chalk, or dry erase board and markers

4. Meal Planning: Variety and Mixed Dishes

SECTION 4.1: VARIETY

This section focuses on reviewing variety among food groups and why we should eat from all the food groups for good health. It also emphasizes that planning a meal ahead of time can increase variety at a meal.

Key Points:

- It is important to eat a variety of foods every day, which means eating foods from several food groups at every meal.
- We need to eat different kinds of foods at each meal because each food has different vitamins. By eating foods from all food groups, we can get all the vitamins we need to be healthy.
- One way to make sure you get enough variety at every meal is to plan your meals ahead of time.

1. Set up three different plates (either photos or actual plates and food models): Meal 1: Chicken, Meal 2: Chicken and rice, Meal 3: Chicken, rice, and vegetables.
2. Ask the students to look at the 3 plates and name the food group(s) that they see on each one.
3. Ask them, "Which plate is the healthiest? Why did you choose that one?"
4. Explain that meal 3 is the healthiest because it has 3 different food groups in it.
5. Remind the students that the word **variety** (hold up flashcard) means eating foods from all the different food groups, and that we should do this at every meal. Explain that we need to eat different kinds of foods at each meal because each kind of food has different **vitamins** (hold up flashcard). By eating foods from all the food groups, we can get all the vitamins we need to be healthy.
6. Explain that one way to increase variety is to plan your meals ahead of time, to make sure they include all of the food groups.

LESSON TIPS

✓ If mixed dishes come up, tell students you'll be talking about them next.

✓ Use food pictures and models to come up with additional "variety" meals.

At this point in the lesson, transition into Activity 4.1. For students who have already completed the "brown bag lunch" activity in Lesson 1, repeat as needed, or make it more complicated by providing lunches missing 2 or more food groups.

ACTIVITY 4.1: LEVEL 1, KNOWLEDGE-CENTERED ACTIVITY

In this "brown bag lunch" game, students will search pre-made bagged lunches containing 4 items. Each item is from a specific food group but one food group is missing. The students must identify the missing food group. This activity will help students practice their food categorizing skills and reinforce the concept of variety.

1. One at a time, each student empties a bagged lunch and determines which food group is missing. Encourage the student to use the 5 food group cards to identify which food groups are in the lunch in order to find the missing one.
2. The student then completes the meal by choosing a food from the missing group.
3. Repeat these steps until each student has had a turn.

Alternate activity: Have students construct a healthy lunch by choosing foods from assorted pictures or food models, emphasizing that they choose one food from each food group.

SECTION 4.2: MIXED DISHES

This section focuses on mixed dishes, which are foods or meals with more than one food group combined; as a result, it can be difficult to tease apart which food groups are represented. This section relies heavily on visual and manual examples that pull apart mixed dishes into their respective food groups.

Key Points:
- "Mixed dishes" are foods that contain more than one food group.
- Mixed dishes can be a great way to get variety but are often low in vegetables, so it's important to find ways to add them in.

Note: Have Activity 4.2A set up and refer to it during this lesson.

1. Hold up the pizza slice (Appendix L) and ask students, "What food group is pizza in?" (This is a tricky question.)
2. Tell students that the piece of pizza has three food groups in it, and that we call a food like this a "mixed dish" because it has more than one food group in it.
3. Ask students if they can tell you why there are 3 food groups in pizza and which ones they are. Show students that the 3 parts of the pizza are crust, sauce, and cheese and pull it apart.
4. Use frozen dinner boxes or photos from a magazine to show students additional examples of mixed dishes. Ask students to look at each part of the dish and figure out its food group.
5. Ask them what they could add to the meal to make it healthier.
6. Explain that mixed dishes can be a great way to get variety, but often they don't have enough vegetables or fruits, so it's important to add them in as much as possible.
7. Ask students again if they have other ideas about how they could add more vegetables or fruits to the pizza to make it a healthier meal.

At this point in the lesson, have students attempt their own mixed dishes in Activity 4.2.

ACTIVITY 4.2A: LEVELS 1 & 2, KNOWLEDGE-CENTERED ACTIVITY

In this activity, students will identify all the food groups in a mixed dish and add food(s) to the dish to increase variety and complete the meal.

1. Give a student a mixed dish to pull apart into pieces and match pieces to the correct food group column. Correct as needed.
2. Talk about which food groups are missing from the mixed dish and ask students to complete the meal by adding in food(s) from the missing groups.
3. Continue with each mixed dish until each student has a turn.

ACTIVITY TIPS

✓Encourage class discussion and participation.

✓Encourage fruits and veggies to complete the meal!

ACTIVITY 4.2B: LEVEL 2, SKILL-CENTERED ACTIVITY

As a group, the class will plan a meal and write a shopping list.

1. Write "What are we eating for dinner?" across the top of the board. Ask students to come up with ideas for dinner meals and let students vote for their favorite option.
2. Using the chosen meal, write "Shopping List" on the board. Support students in naming all required ingredients for the meal, including those needed for cooking, such as oil or spices.
3. Optional: Depending on the resources and time available, actually prepare the meal.

ACTIVITY TIPS

✓Include all five food groups in the meal.

✓Use visuals and give students ample time to process the information and respond.

✓This can be a very challenging activity, especially if students have never grocery shopped or planned a meal before.

✓If you make the meal, choose foods that can be independently prepared, such as frozen or pre-chopped vegetables, and microwavable foods.

"KEEP MOVING"

Take 15 minutes at the end of class to participate in an interactive physical activity (see Appendix F for ideas).

PHYSICAL ACTIVITY TIP
In keeping with the theme of variety, have student do three different cardio exercises for five minutes each.

If resources are available, try to conclude each lesson with a taste test. Taste test ideas:

- **Tuna fish salad with chopped vegetables mixed in, topped with melted low-fat cheese on crackers**
- **English muffin pizzas topped with low fat cheese and vegetables**

TASTE TEST TIP
Prepare what you can and set up the taste test while students are participating in the physical activity. Let students assemble the test taste

DAILY WRAP-UP (Appendix E)

Add vegetables to a mixed dish that you're eating this week. For example, put peppers on your pizza, broccoli in your macaroni and cheese, or mixed vegetables into your casserole.

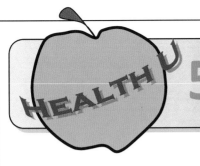

OVERVIEW

In this lesson, students will learn about why they should limit added sugar and how to identify foods with added sugar. It precedes lessons about making healthy choices in general, as added sugar is a complex topic. This lesson integrates activities into the lecture due to the advanced nature of the concepts and skills presented.

LEARNING OBJECTIVES

At the end of the session, students will be able to:
- ✓ Explain why it is not healthy to eat or drink foods that are high in added sugar
- ✓ Identify food and drinks with and without added sugar, either by reading the front label or the nutrition facts

MATERIALS AND PREPARATION

<u>General Materials for the Lesson</u>
Appendix Materials
- Flashcard for vitamins (Appendix A)
- Fruit food group card (Appendix B)
- Printed photographs of individual fruits (Appendix C)
- "Take Home Ideas" worksheet (Appendix E)
- Physical activity ideas (Appendix F)

Additional Materials (see Guidelines for Use, p. iii, for tips on obtaining these)
- Additional images and food models of foods with and without added sugar: soda, seltzer, plain and sweetened yogurt and milk, candy, fruit snacks, muffins, cookies, ice cream

5. Added Sugars

MATERIALS AND PREPARATION

Activity-Specific Materials and Preparation

Activity 5.1

Materials

Appendix Materials – None

Additional Materials

- 12-ounce can of soda
- Additional sweetened beverages and snacks (i.e., 20-oz bottle of soda, sports drink, fruit drink) with the number of teaspoons of sugar written on the bottom for reference (see equivalents below)
- Fruit snacks
- 1-quart picture of water
- 16-ounce clear plastic or glass cup
- Small paper cups, one per student
- 1 box of sugar packets
- Clear plastic bags
- Funnel
- Spoon

Reminder:

1 teaspoon = 4 grams = 1 sugar packet or cube

20-oz soda/iced tea/fruit drink: 16 tsp sugar

20-oz sports drink: 9-10 tsp sugar

5. Added Sugars

MATERIALS AND PREPARATION

<u>Activity-Specific Materials and Preparation</u>
<u>Activity 5.2A</u>
Materials
Appendix Materials
- Flashcards for: 100% juice; sugar, syrup, fructose (Appendix A)

Additional Materials
- Additional images and real foods or food containers of the following pairs of food:
  > fruit cups packed in 100% juice and fruit cups packed in syrup
  > "no sugar added" (or "natural") apple sauce and "original" apple sauce
  > seltzer and soda
  > sweetened and unsweetened cereal
  > bag of sliced apples and apple-flavored candy

Preparation
1. Tips on choosing items for this lesson:
    - Use only food models that have vocabulary words obviously displayed on the front of the package.
    - Use commonly consumed foods.

<u>Activity 5.2B</u>
Materials
Appendix Materials
- Flashcard for sugar, syrup, fructose (Appendix A)

Additional Materials
- Additional images and models of pairs of food from Activity 5.2A

Preparation
1. This activity is optional dependent on the skills of the students. If you choose to use it, make a poster for your class highlighting what to look for on the nutrition facts label for added sugars.

SECTION 5.1: ADDED SUGAR

This section covers foods that contain added sugar and the reasons for limiting these foods. The lecture is very brief.

Key Points:
- Sugar has energy but no vitamins, so when we eat foods with a lot of sugar, we're not getting what our bodies need.
- Fruit is a good way to eat something sweet-tasting while also getting the vitamins we need.

1. Ask the students, "What foods have a lot of sugar?" Give them the hint to think about foods that taste sweet.
2. Explain that there are lots of drinks, desserts, candy, fruit snacks, and breakfast cereals that contain a lot of sugar.
3. Ask students to give reasons why we should not eat a lot of sugar.
4. Tell students that sugar has energy but no **vitamins** (hold up flashcard), so when we eat foods with a lot of sugar, we're not getting what our bodies need. Also tell students that eating a lot of sugar might cause cavities.
5. Ask, "What foods taste sweet but have *natural* sugar?" (That is, sugar is not added to them.)
6. Tell students that fruit has natural sugar and also has lots of vitamins to keep us healthy.

L E S S O N   T I P S

✓ Rely heavily on pictures and models of foods with and without added sugar.

✓ Include as many foods with added sugar as possible to reinforce the learning objective.

✓ Encourage discussion and interaction.

✓ Discuss foods students consume regularly, especially ones they may not think have added sugar (e.g., fruit drinks and fast food smoothies).

At this point in the lesson, transition into the activity.

ACTIVITY 5.1: LEVEL 1, KNOWLEDGE-CENTERED ACTIVITY

This activity visually demonstrates the added sugar in foods.

1. Pour 12 ounces of water into a cup. Put the materials on a table where all students have a clear view. Have individual sugar packets ready to count out.
2. Pass around the can of soda and glass of water. Tell students that they have the same amount of liquid. Pass around a sugar packet so they know how much is in one.
3. Ask students to guess how many packets of sugar are in one 12-ounce soda (answer: 10 packets).
4. Count out 10 packets of sugar with the students, and have them pour the sugar into the cup of water and stir until the sugar is dissolved.
5. Pour a small cup of the sweetened water for each student to taste so they can describe how sweet it is.
6. Move on to guessing the number of packets in other drinks.

ACTIVITY TIPS

✓ If time is limited, measure sugar ahead of time and have students pour sugar out of bags.

✓ Talk about how at first you see the sugar at the bottom, but after stirring, you can't see it because it dissolves into the liquid. This means that it's often hard to tell how much sugar is in the drink once the sugar is mixed in.

✓ Choose foods based on student preferences, such as (unsweetened) iced tea, lemonade, fast food smoothies or slushies, cereal, candy, popsicles, pudding, and Jell-O.

✓ Choose some items that have a lot of sugar (e.g., a 32-oz smoothie or frozen coffee drink), as it can be surprising how much sugar is in them!

✓ If students are having trouble guessing the numbers of packets, put a certain number in front of the drink or food and use the words "more" or "enough" so that they can guess that way. For example, a 20-oz soda has 16 packets of sugar in it. Start with 10 packets and ask the students if they think that's enough or there is more sugar in the drink. Keep adding packets until the students think there is enough.

SECTION 5.2: HEALTHIER SWEET CHOICES

This section teaches the healthiest alternatives to sweetened food and drinks and emphasizes the important of eating whole fruit.

Key Points:

- It's important not to eat too much added sugar. There are healthier choices you can make and still have foods that taste sweet.
- If consuming fruit juice, it should be 100% juice and be limited to 4 ounces per day.
- Fruit is a great way to add a sweet taste to your food, because it has lots of vitamins.

1. Explain to students that it's important not to eat too much added sugar, and that there are healthier choices they can make and still have foods that taste sweet.
2. Show students the flashcard for **100% juice** and explain what it means. Explain that they can look for drinks that say 100% juice on the label to know there is no sugar added to those drinks.
3. Ask students to think of some healthy drinks that don't have any added sugar.
4. Ask, "What about cereals? Can you think of any cereals that taste very sweet?" Once the students have given some ideas, ask, "What could you add to cereal to make it taste sweet without adding sugar?"
5. Tell students they could slice a banana or strawberries into cereal, or add raisins or Craisins (dried cranberry). Explain that fruit is a great way to add a sweet taste to your food, because it has lots of vitamins to keep us healthy.
6. Ask students what food group they could have for dessert instead of foods with added sugar.

L E S S O N   T I P S

✓ Keep the discussion very short and integrate the activity and visuals throughout as needed.

✓ Use materials from previous lessons to remind students of the wide variety of fruits available.

✓ Rely heavily on pictures and food models to encourage students to come up with examples on their own.

✓ Students may suggest fruit and sports drinks as healthy choices; remind them again that these have added sugar.

At this point in the lesson, transition into activity 5.2A for practice reading the front package on food products. For more advanced students who master this concept quickly, move forward and use Activity 5.2B.

ACTIVITY 5.2A: LEVEL 1, SKILL-CENTERED ACTIVITY

In this activity, students will practice reading food packages to find foods without added sugar.

1. Set up a display of several pairs of food items on a large table.
2. Have students examine the two food items in each pair to figure out which one doesn't have added sugar, and ask students to choose which one of the two is the healthier choice to buy.
3. Repeat for all food pairs.

A note on sugar substitutes:
This can be a very complicated subject! Some students' parents may have told them to only drink diet drinks, whereas other families may avoid sugar substitutes altogether. Depending on your students, you may want to discuss the pros and cons of sugar substitutes. Use your discretion, and look into current medical and nutritional science literature for advice.

> **ACTIVITY TIP**
>
> ✓ Review flashcards as foods are introduced.

Discussion points using population-appropriate language:
Sugar substitutes may not have any energy or calories in them, but some scientists are beginning to question whether they are a healthy choice. The *best* drinks to choose are water, seltzer, milk, and unsweetened tea and coffee. If you choose drinks with a sugar substitute, it's best not to have too many of them each day.

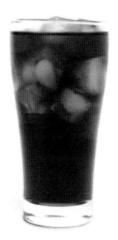 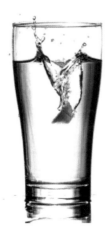

ACTIVITY 5.2B: LEVEL 2, SKILL-CENTERED ACTIVITY (Optional)

Students will practice finding unsweetened options and learn how to read the nutritional facts panel and ingredients list.

1. Show the students the **sugar, syrup, fructose** flashcard and explain that they can look for these words in an ingredients list to find out whether that food has added sugar.
2. Ask students to come up and look at one of the pairs of items to figure out which one has added sugar based on the ingredients list.
3. Next, explain that we can also find out how much sugar a food has based on looking at the nutrition facts label on the package. Show them where to find "Sugars" on the label.
4. Ask students to come up and look at the pairs of items to figure out which one has the smallest amount of sugar by looking at the "Sugars" amount on the nutrition facts label.

L E S S O N   T I P S

✓This is an advanced-topic lesson. Identifying these words isn't vital for understanding the concept of added sugars, but may help if students are independent grocery shoppers. Only use this lesson as needed.

✓Ingredients and nutrition facts can be very difficult to read because of the font size. Make blown-up copies of the label to pass around.

✓Choose items with the same or similar serving sizes as much as possible. Ensure that the amount of "sugar" is highest in the sweetened item.

✓The concept of "less than" and "more than" can be difficult, while "smaller" and "bigger" are easier to grasp.

"KEEP MOVING"

Take 15 minutes at the end of class to participate in an interactive physical activity (see Appendix F for ideas).

PHYSICAL ACTIVITY TIP

Encourage students to be more active by taking the stairs instead of the elevator or encouraging their parents to park the car farther away from where they are going.

If resources are available, try to conclude each lesson with a taste test. Taste test ideas:

Juice cocktail: 1 part 100% juice to 2 parts seltzer

TASTE TEST TIP

Include a "recipe" slip with this taste test, along with a reminder of beverages to replace soda: water, sparkling water/seltzer, milk, and 100% juice.

DAILY WRAP-UP (Appendix E)

Try a new fruit this week.

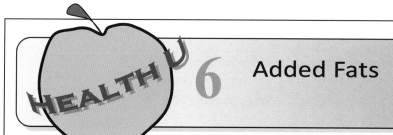

HEALTH U 6 Added Fats

OVERVIEW

This lesson focuses on fats and reviews those cooking methods that do and do not add fat, as well as healthy choices for condiments. The lesson also teaches the differences among grilled, steamed, and fried foods and the implications of each.

LEARNING OBJECTIVES

At the end of the session, students will be able to:
- ✓ Name high-fat and low-fat cooking methods
- ✓ Explain why fried foods should be limited
- ✓ Find lower-fat options for spreads and dressings
- ✓ Differentiate between healthy and unhealthy fats

MATERIALS AND PREPARATION

General Materials for the Lesson

Appendix Materials
- Flashcards with each of the following terms on one side, and the definition on the other: grilled, baked, steamed, fried, light/lite, low or reduced fat, fat free (Appendix A)
- "Take Home Ideas" worksheet (Appendix E)
- Physical activity ideas (Appendix F)

Additional Materials (see Guidelines for Use, p. iii, for tips on obtaining these)
- Pictures of the following: fried and grilled chicken, French fries and baked potato, steamed and deep-fried mushrooms, microwaved and fried broccoli, salad with dressing on it versus salad with dressing on the side. Label each picture. Choose images where it is obvious that the item is fried versus steamed, baked, microwaved, or grilled.
- Videos or pictures of the following cooking techniques: baking, grilling, steaming, microwaving, frying
- 2 bottles of salad dressing, one regular, one light; pictures of butter and oil. Choose items that are very similar-looking: same-sized salads, same types of dressing, so their differences are obvious.
- 2 small containers: one with 2 tablespoons oil (labeled "regular") and one with 2 teaspoons oil (labeled "light")

6.   Added Fats

MATERIALS AND PREPARATION

Activity-Specific Materials and Preparation

<u>Activity 6.1</u>
Materials
Appendix Materials – None
Additional Materials
- 1 slice of white bread on a small plate
- 1 tablespoon + 1 teaspoon of oil, in a leak-proof container

<u>Activity 6.2</u>
Materials
Appendix Materials
- Flashcards with each of the following terms on one side, and the definition on the other: light/lite, low or reduced fat, fat free (Appendix A)

Additional Materials
- Plastic food models and/or real food or food containers of the following: reduced fat and regular mayonnaise, light and regular dressing, light and regular butter, low fat and regular sour cream, fat free and regular cream cheese
  - Tips for selecting foods:
    - Use only food models that have vocabulary words obviously displayed on the front of the food package.
    - Use typically consumed foods.

SECTION 6.1: HEALTHY COOKING/
ACTIVITY 6.1: LEVEL 1, KNOWLEDGE-CENTERED ACTIVITY

This section exposes students to different cooking preparations and explains why it is important to choose the healthier food (steamed, microwaved, grilled) over fried foods.

Key Points:

- It's important to choose grilled, baked, steamed, or microwaved foods instead of fried foods to be healthy.
- Limit fried foods because they are cooked in oil, which is a type of fat. The oil gets soaked up by the food, so we end up eating a lot of it.

Note: Because Activity 6.1 takes time, it is incorporated here as part of the lecture. This activity visually demonstrates the amount of fat that is added to food while it is fried.

1. Pass around the oil (1 Tbs + 1 tsp, in a leak-proof container) and explain to students that it's how much oil you would eat in most large-size French fries at a fast food restaurant.
2. Explain that most fried food is breaded (use the pictures of fried mushrooms and nuggets), so the bread soaks up the oil while the food cooks. Explain that French fries don't need to be breaded because the potato is really good at soaking up the oil.
3. Ask a student to pour the oil over the bread and set it aside while the bread soaks up the oil (15-20 minutes).
4. Ask students if they know any different ways to cook a certain food (for example, chicken). If they give a variety of answers, ask whether they have any thoughts on which ways are considered healthier.
5. Explain that there are certain ways of cooking foods that are healthy because they do not add any oil, butter, or other fat to the food in order to cook it.

LESSON TIPS

✓ Videos are the best way to demonstrate cooking methods, especially since these methods may be new to students.

✓ Promote microwaving as a method students can use independently. Describe it as very similar to steaming and focus on it as a low-fat cooking technique they can do on their own.

✓ It is vital for students to be able to recognize vocabulary terms (baked, steamed, grilled, or fried), visually or verbally, so they can make the healthiest choices.

✓ Each time fried foods come up in the discussion, reiterate that they are something to limit.

SECTION 6.1: HEALTHY COOKING/
ACTIVITY 6.1: LEVEL 1, KNOWLEDGE-CENTERED ACTIVITY (continued)

6. Hold up 2 pictures of the same food, cooked 2 different ways. Ask the students which one is healthier, and why. Use this as a way to introduce the various vocabulary terms from the lesson.
7. Hold up the pictures of fried and grilled chicken. Explain that **grilled** (hold up flashcard) foods are healthier than fried foods because they are grilled over a fire with no added fat. Show the students the grill marks (black lines) on the chicken and explain that that's one way to know if a food has been grilled.
8. Hold up the pictures of a baked potato and French fries. Ask the students which one is healthier. Explain that the baked potato is the healthier choice because **baked** (hold up flashcard) foods are cooked in the oven with no added fat.
9. Hold up the pictures of steamed versus breaded and fried mushrooms. Ask which one is healthier. Explain that the steamed mushrooms are healthier because **steamed** (hold up flashcard) foods are cooked with a little bit of water below them, and you don't need to add any fat. Tell the students that you can also use the microwave to steam foods.
10. Last, ask the students to look at all of the fried foods. Explain that **fried** (hold up flashcard) foods are cooked in oil, which is a type of fat. Because the oil gets soaked up by the food, we end up eating a lot of it, which means we're eating a lot of fat.
11. Emphasize that it's important to choose grilled, baked, steamed, or microwaved foods instead of fried ones to be healthy.
12. Discuss the differences in the way the foods look and taste depending on how they're cooked (fried tastes crunchy and salty, while the others usually taste more fresh).
13. After 15-20 minutes, hold up the bread and show how it glistens. Note that the oil is soaked up by the bread and there is no longer a pool of oil on top.

SECTION 6.2: FATS AND OILS

This section is about fats in condiments – sauces, dips, dressings, and spreads – and presents ways to limit fats.

Key Points:
- When eating out, order sauces and dips on the side.
- Some liquid oils are healthier than solid fats like butter.
- Look for light salad dressings in the grocery store.

1. Ask the students, "What are some of your favorite sauces or dressings?"
2. Explain that in this section, we're going to talk about all of these things (the condiments they list) because they can have a lot of fat in them, and it's important to limit fat when you're trying to eat healthy because too much fat is not good for your heart.
3. Show students a picture of a salad with dressing on it and a salad with dressing on the side. Ask them which one is healthier, and why.
4. Explain that both salads are a *great* way to eat lots of vegetables, but salad dressing can have a lot of fat in it. It's healthier to order salad dressing on the side, and use only a very small amount to start out. Most restaurants give you much more dressing than you actually need.
5. Next, show the students two bottles of dressing – one regular and one light – and ask them which one is healthier and why. Explain that **light/lite** (hold up flashcard) dressings have much less fat than regular dressings. Pass around the 2 containers of oil (one holding 2 Tbs and labeled "regular", one holding 2 tsp and labeled "light") to show how much fat is in regular dressing.
6. Next, show the students photos of butter and oil. Ask them which is healthier. If students aren't sure, reassure them that it's a tricky one. Explain that liquid fats like oils are better for us than solid fats like butter because oils are much healthier for our hearts. However, remind them we still want to limit the amount.
7. Explain that food packaging can often tell us how much fat a food has. Look for foods that say **light/lite, low or reduced fat**, and **fat free** (hold up flashcard for each term).

LESSON TIPS

✓Have Activity 6.2 set up in advance of the lesson and refer to it so students can see examples of condiments.

✓Hold up food models, pictures, and vocabulary terms as they are discussed.

At this point in the lesson, transition into Activity 6.2.

ACTIVITY 6.2: LEVEL 1, SKILL-CENTERED ACTIVITY

In this activity, students will practice finding low-fat options based on food packaging.

1. Display food packages in pairs on a large table.
2. Have students examine the pairs one at a time. Using the flash cards for the words **light/lite, low or reduced fat,** and **fat free**, have students figure out which item in the pair is healthier to buy.
3. Repeat for all pairs.

ACTIVITY TIP

✓This activity can also be done using an online grocer or at the grocery store. Be sure to bring the flashcards to use as a resource while online shopping or at the grocery store.

"KEEP MOVING"

Take 15 minutes at the end of class to participate in an interactive physical activity (see Appendix F for ideas).

PHYSICAL ACTIVITY TIP

At this point, students have completed more than half of the program. Ask students to do a physical activity instead of watching a TV show.

If resources are available, try to conclude each lesson with a taste test. Taste test ideas:

- **Cut vegetables with light ranch dip**
- **Pieces of grilled chicken marinated in light salad dressing (prepare in advance)**

TASTE TEST TIP

Encourage students to discuss healthy cooking methods with their parents by having them write it on their Take Home Ideas sheet (Appendix E).

DAILY WRAP-UP (Appendix E)

Try eating steamed or grilled food this week.

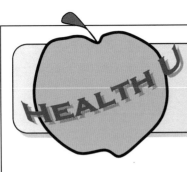

7 Making Healthy Choices

OVERVIEW

In this lesson, students will learn how to make the healthiest choices within each food group, based on their background knowledge of the food groups and the need to limit fat and sugar. This lesson is organized somewhat differently, in that the activity is integrated throughout the lesson as each food group is discussed.

LEARNING OBJECTIVES

At the end of the session, students will be able to:
- ✓ Explain the importance and health benefits of whole grains, low-fat dairy, and lean meat
- ✓ Compare food choices and pick the healthiest choice
- ✓ Modify less healthy meals by substituting food items for healthier versions

MATERIALS AND PREPARATION

<u>General Materials for the Lesson</u>
Appendix Materials
- Flashcards from lessons 5 and 6 (added sugar, added fat) to review as necessary (Appendix A)
- 5 food group cards (Appendix B)
- Printed photographs of individual foods, representing all 5 food groups (Appendix C)
- "Take Home Ideas" worksheet (Appendix E)
- Physical activity ideas (Appendix F)
- Handout of "Switch-A-Roo Ideas" for students to take home (Appendix M)

Additional Materials (see Guidelines for Use, p. iii, for tips on obtaining these)
- Food models of whole and fat-free milk, plain and sweetened yogurt
- Pictures of the following: marbleized meat, meat with fat on the edges, meat trimmed of fat; salami and bacon with visible white fat throughout; chicken and turkey with and without skin; fish; veggie burger; egg; beans; peanut butter

7. Making Healthy Choices

MATERIALS AND PREPARATION

Activity-Specific Materials and Preparation
Activity 7.1
Materials
Appendix Materials
- Laminated pictures of healthy and un-healthy food items (Appendix M)
  - Note: Modify meals and pantry items to students' cultural and dietary habits.

Additional Materials
- Corkboard with push pins
- Tri-fold foam core poster board
- Small box or bin
- Note: This activity can alternately be done with Velcro and felt board. Tape also works well, but the transition between meals is much slower, and it limits how easy the foods are to maneuver.

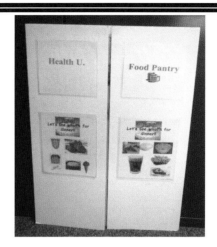

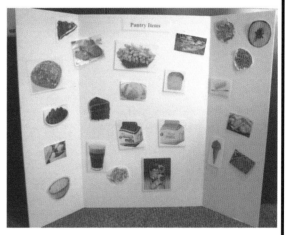

Preparation
1. Arrange one meal at a time on the corkboard with four or five unhealthy choices.
   - Meal 1: Breakfast: bacon, high-sugar cereal, whole milk, sugary drink
   - Meal 2: Lunch: hot dog, white bread, fries, pie, soda
   - Meal 3: Dinner: fried chicken, fried vegetables, white pasta, cream sauce, ice cream
   - Meal 4: Dinner: fish nuggets, chips, chocolate cupcake, white rice, butter
2. Attach healthy and unhealthy food items inside the tri-fold board with Velcro or tape. Be sure to include the healthy items that will be substituted for the unhealthy food items already on the corkboard for that specific meal.
3. Close the tri-fold board and label the outside "Pantry."
4. Label the small box or bin "No Thank You Bin."

ACTIVITY 7.1: LEVEL 1, KNOWLEDGE-CENTERED ACTIVITY

In this "Switch-A-Roo for Healthy Food" activity, students make meal substitutions. First, students are presented with an unhealthy meal, and they are then offered a number of foods from the "Pantry" to choose a healthy substitution.

1. Ask the students if the meal on the corkboard is healthy. Explain that they're going to use the pantry to learn how to make it healthier.
2. Start with a grain, vegetable, or fruit, as they have already learned how to make healthy choices in this group.
3. Ask a student to remove one of the unhealthy foods from the meal on the board and place it in the "No Thank You Bin." Have them look in the pantry for a healthier item to replace the unhealthy one. During this process, review how to make healthy choices within that specific food group. (Use Section 7.1 below as a review for grains, fruit, and vegetables.)
4. Check the student's substitution and ask them to explain why their choice is healthier.
5. Repeat steps 3 and 4 with the remaining food groups.
6. Continue with dairy and protein foods. Use Section 7.2 to cover new material on how to make healthy dairy and protein choices.
7. Repeat with other meals as time allows.

ACTIVITY TIPS

✓ Healthy substitutions should stay in the same group.

✓ For an easier option, only fill the pantry with one food group at a time.

SECTION 7.1: REVIEW OF HEALTH CHOICES FOR GRAINS, VEGETABLES, & FRUITS

Key Points:

- Choose whole grains instead of white grains. One way to figure out if a grain is whole is to look for a brown color.
- Choose whole fruits and canned fruits with no added sugar instead of canned fruits in syrup, fruit snacks, and gummy treats.
- Choose fresh/raw, steamed, boiled, baked, or microwaved vegetables instead of fried vegetables or French fries.

1. Use the activity itself to guide the delivery of the key points above. As students come up, ask them, "Is there a healthier [grain/fruit/vegetable] in the pantry?"
2. Ask them, "How do we know it's healthier?"

LESSON TIPS

✓Use the corresponding food group card when discussing that group.

✓Substitutions should be made within the same food group; for example, substitute grilled chicken for fried chicken, substitute brown rice for white, and so forth.

✓Spend the most time on new concepts, but if students are confused, use flashcards and review materials from lessons 1-6.

Activity 7.1 will continue and take place simultaneously with Section 7.2.

SECTION 7.2: HEALTHY CHOICES FOR DAIRY & PROTEIN/ ACTIVITY 7.1: LEVEL 1, KNOWLEDGE-CENTERED ACTIVITY (continued)

This section introduces the concept that the healthiest dairy choices are low-fat and unsweetened, and that the healthiest proteins are lean or come from plants.

Key Points:
- Low fat and unsweetened dairy are the healthiest dairy choices.
- The healthiest proteins are lean (fish, chicken, turkey) or come from plants, including beans and nuts.

1. Show the students three cartons of milk, one whole, one 1%, and one skim. Ask them what the differences are between them and which one is healthiest. Explain that the carton of whole milk has a lot of fat, the carton of 1% milk has a little bit of fat, and the carton of fat-free milk has no fat. Another name for fat-free milk is skim milk.
2. Ask the students, "Why don't we want to eat too much fat?" Remind students that too much fat is bad for our hearts, so it's best to choose fat-free and reduced-fat dairy.
3. Next, show the students two containers of yogurt, one plain (unsweetened) and one sweetened. Ask them which one is healthier. Explain that one yogurt is plain, and the other has sugar added, not real fruit.
4. Ask the students why we don't want to eat a lot of sugar. Remind students that too much sugar is bad for our teeth, and it doesn't have any extra vitamins. It's healthier to choose plain yogurt and add real fruit instead of sugar to make it taste sweet.
5. Now ask the students, "Is ice cream the healthiest dairy to pick?" Explain that because ice cream has both added fat *and* sugar, it is not the healthiest dairy.

At this point in the lesson, have the students switch-a-roo the dairy in meal 1.

LESSON TIPS

✓ Hold up food models, pictures, and vocabulary terms as they are discussed in each food group. Pass them around for a closer look.

✓ Introduce new food concepts before asking them to make a healthy substitution.

✓ Review added fat and sugar as needed.

✓ Review these concepts as needed when additional Switch-A-Roo meals are introduced.

SECTION 7.2: HEALTHY CHOICES FOR DAIRY & PROTEIN/ ACTIVITY 7.1: LEVEL 1, KNOWLEDGE-CENTERED ACTIVITY (continued)

1. Explain that next we're going to look at the protein part of the meal.
2. Show the students the pictures of steak. Ask them which one is healthier. Explain that, in one picture, the white part on the edges and swirling through the meat is fat. In another picture, the fat has been trimmed off. It's important to choose meat that has very little white fat in it.
3. Next, show the pictures of bacon and salami. Ask the students what they notice. Explain that there is a lot of white in both of them, which means they have a lot of fat.
4. Move on to the chicken and turkey. Again ask students what they notice, and explain that all of the fat is in the skin. If you take the skin off, these meats have no fat on them.
5. Next, show the pictures of the fish and veggie burger. Ask what the students notice, and point out that we can't see any white fat in these two, so they are very healthy.
6. Ask students, "What about eggs, beans, and nuts? Are these healthy proteins?" Tell students that beans and nuts are very healthy types of proteins. Beans are low in fat and have a lot of fiber, and nuts have healthy fats in them.

Now switch-a-roo the protein in meal 1.

Then continue with meals 2-4 and focus on reviewing healthy choices within *each* food group. Dairy and protein will likely need the most review, as these are new concepts.

"KEEP MOVING"

Take 15 minutes at the end of class to participate in an interactive physical activity (see Appendix F for ideas).

PHYSICAL ACTIVITY TIP

Create a sheet describing the activities the students have participated in thus far. Give one to each student and have them circle or star their favorites.

If resources are available, try to conclude each lesson with a taste test. Taste test ideas:

- **Reduced-fat cheese with whole-wheat crackers**
- **Low-fat plain yogurt with sliced fruit**

TASTE TEST TIP

Use this taste test as a teaching opportunity. Show students the label from the yogurt or cheese and have them find vocabulary words that show that they are healthy foods in the dairy group.

DAILY WRAP-UP (Appendix E)

Try one of the substitutions on the "Switch-A-Roo Ideas" handout (Appendix M).

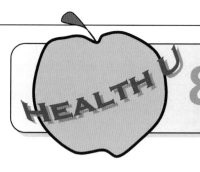

Healthy Snacks vs. Treats

8

OVERVIEW

This lesson covers the topic of healthy snacking choices. Since there is very little new material in this lesson, use it as an opportunity to assess what the students have learned about the concepts covered thus far. Review previous concepts such as the five food groups, added sugar, and added fats as needed.

LEARNING OBJECTIVES

At the end of the session, students will be able to:
- ✓ Define healthy snack
- ✓ Describe healthy snack choices and when to eat snacks
- ✓ Describe what makes a food a "treat"

MATERIALS AND PREPARATION

General Materials for the Lesson

Appendix Materials
- 5 food group cards (Appendix B)
- Printed photographs of individual foods, representing all five food groups (Appendix C)
- Vocabulary flashcards to review as needed (Appendix A)
- "Take Home Ideas" worksheet (Appendix E)
- Physical activity ideas (Appendix F)

Additional Materials (see Guidelines for Use, p. iii, for tips on obtaining these)
- Food models and pictures of healthy snacks from each food group, as well as dessert, candy, and other treats that don't fit into food groups

8.   Healthy Snacks vs. Treats

MATERIALS AND PREPARATION

Activity-Specific Materials and Preparation

Activity 8.1

Materials

Appendix Materials

- 2x3" playing cards (Appendix N):
    - 27 pairs of healthy snack cards
    - 9 treat cards (*Note:* These intentionally do not have a pair.)

Additional Materials

- Small bucket or box labeled "treat bucket"

Activity 8.2

Materials

Appendix Materials

- Jerseys (*add student names*), cut out and laminated (Appendix O)
- Score board, cut out and laminated (Appendix O)
- Sample snack cards for students to take home (Appendix O)
    - 1-point snack: any snack that fits into the grain, dairy, or protein food group
    - 2-point snack: any snack with a fruit or vegetable

Additional Materials

- Dry erase marker

SECTION 8.1: HEALTHY SNACKS VS. TREATS

This section discusses snacks, or food eaten between meals, and how to differentiate between healthy snacks and treats.

Key Points:
- Healthy snacks fit into one of the five food groups.
- Healthy snacks can help if you are hungry between meals, or if you exercise a lot and need more energy.
- Treats like dessert and candy are not healthy snacks because they have a lot of fat and sugar but no vitamins.

1. Put out a variety of healthy snacks and treats on a table and ask, "Do you see any food on the table that might be a healthy snack?"
2. Once the students have selected a few options, ask them how they know those options are healthy. Explain that healthy snacks fit into one of the five food groups (review concepts from lessons 1-6 as needed).
3. Ask the students, "When is it a good time to snack?" Explain that healthy snacks can help when you're hungry between meals, or if you exercise a lot and need more energy, but you don't *always* need a snack.
4. Pick up a dessert or candy, and ask, "What about this? Is it a healthy snack?"
5. Explain that the dessert/candy is a treat, not a healthy snack. It has a lot of fat and sugar, but no vitamins. It's fine to have desserts and candy sometimes, but you don't need them every day.
6. Ask the students if they see anything on the table they could have instead of the dessert/candy.
7. Have the students come up to the table and point out healthy snacks and treats. Practice making healthy snacks using food pictures or models.
8. If you would like to focus on variety, teach students to choose snacks with at least two food groups.

LESSON TIPS

✓Use a wide variety of food models and pictures for both treats and healthy snacks.

✓This lesson has very little new material. Use it as an opportunity to assess what the students have learned thus far and to review concepts that are not well understood.

✓Reiterate which foods are treats and which are healthy choices.

At this point in the lesson, transition into Activity 8.1.

ACTIVITY 8.1: LEVEL 1, KNOWLEDGE-CENTERED ACTIVITY

In "Go Snack," students will play a fun and interactive card game based on "Go Fish."

Rules (similar to the card game "Go Fish"):
Each student receives a hand of cards. The object is to get rid of all the cards in your hand by finding pairs of healthy snacks. When a healthy snack pair is found, the pair is laid down on the table. Students will ask another player if they have a card in order to obtain a pair. If the card is not in the other student's hand, the first student will need to draw a card from the "Go Snack" center pile.

The tricky part: Foods that are treats do not have pairs! Dispose of the treat in the "treat bucket" instead of trying to find its pair.

1. Explain the rules of the game.
2. Shuffle and deal the playing cards. Ensure there are enough cards for the "Go Snack" pile in the center of the table.
3. One at a time, students put their pairs on the table and their treats in the treat bucket. When they put down a pair, ask them to name the food group.
4. Player 1 will request a food on a card they have in their hand by asking for it from player 2.
    - *If player 2 has the requested snack*, he must hand over the card. Player 1 puts the pair down and names the food group.
    - *If player 2 does not have the requested snack*, player 1 draws from the "Go Snack" pile in the center of the table.
    - *If player 1 names a treat*, review why it is a treat. Player 1 then puts the treat in the treat bucket and chooses from the "Go Snack" pile.
5. The next student repeats step 4.
6. Continue playing until all students get rid of their cards.

ACTIVITY TIPS

✓ The number of cards accommodates 3-6 players comfortably. For larger groups, start a second game with another set of cards.

✓ Use this game to reinforce the idea of healthy snacks.

✓ Encourage the students to pick out their favorites from the healthy snack cards.

✓ For an easier modification, play only with the healthy snack cards and leave out the treats.

✓ No need to have a winner! Play until everyone is done.

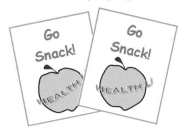

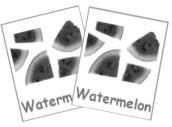

ACTIVITY 8.2: LEVEL 1, KNOWLEDGE-CENTERED ACTIVITY

The goal of this activity is to encourage healthy snacking. This activity can be continued beyond the Health U. lessons by incorporating it into a daily classroom routine.

In this activity, students will earn points for making healthy snack choices at home. Students in the class work as a team to meet a goal for the classroom; they do not compete with each other. The instructor can work with students to set a specific goal based on how often they play the game.

Rules:

Students receive 2 points for any snack that contains a fruit or vegetable; 1 point for a snack that fits into the grain, dairy, or protein food group; and 0 points for treats.

1. Explain the rules of the game.
2. Give students a snack card to take home and have them indicate, either in writing or by pasting a picture, one snack they had yesterday. If class only meets once a week, you can give them a snack card for each day of the week or choose several days.
3. Show the students their laminated jerseys. Explain to them that they will be given points for the number of healthy snacks they had based on their snack card(s). This will be recorded on their jerseys, which will be displayed on a board in the classroom.
4. Set a goal (number of points earned) with the class.
5. When students next return to class:
   a. Collect the snack cards.
   b. Discuss with each student what snacks they had, and help them determine how many points they earned.
   c. With a dry erase marker, write each student's points on his/her jersey.
   d. Tally the total points for the class on the scoreboard.
   e. Post the jerseys on a board in the classroom along with a scoreboard that shows classroom totals.

> **ACTIVITY TIPS**
>
> ✓ Dry erase markers should easily wipe off of laminated items, but test one first!
>
> ✓ For added fun, the classroom can win a prize by meeting their goal.

What snack I had today	
Apple	2 points
Cookie	0 points

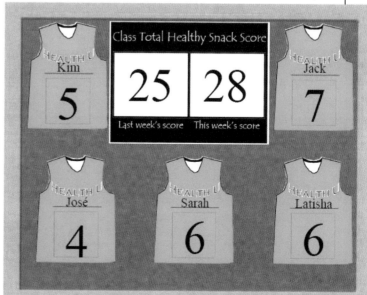

"KEEP MOVING"

Take 15 minutes at the end of class to participate in an interactive physical activity (see Appendix F for ideas).

PHYSICAL ACTIVITY TIP
Encourage students to do their favorite physical activities at home.

If resources are available, try to conclude each lesson with a taste test. Taste test ideas:

- **Cheese and apple slices**
- **Sun butter and celery sticks**
- **Hummus and whole-wheat pita chips**

TASTE TEST TIP
Make a worksheet with healthy snack ideas. Design the worksheet with two columns of food so students can mix and match their own healthy snacks.

DAILY WRAP-UP (Appendix E)

Pack a healthy snack for work or school.

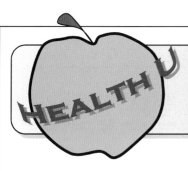

9   Healthy Portions with MyPlate

OVERVIEW

The goal of this lesson is to introduce the MyPlate as a means of choosing the healthiest portions. The optional section of this lesson has students using everyday items to measure snacks and condiments.

LEARNING OBJECTIVES

At the end of the session, students will be able to:
- ✓ Describe healthy portion sizes
- ✓ Measure serving sizes using MyPlate proportions
- ✓ Use MyPlate to assemble a meal with healthy portions

MATERIALS AND PREPARATION

General Materials for the Lesson
Appendix Materials
- Flashcard with healthy portions on one side and the definition on the opposite side (Appendix A)
- 5 food group cards (Appendix B)
- Printed photographs of individual foods, representing all five food groups (Appendix C)
- Image of MyPlate (Appendix D)
- "Take Home Ideas" worksheet (Appendix E)
- Physical activity ideas (Appendix F)

Additional Materials (see Guidelines for Use, p. iii, for tips on obtaining these)
- Additional images of food items from each food group
- Large (at least 27" x 39") poster representation of MyPlate
- *Optional:* Ping pong ball, deck of cards, tennis ball
- *Optional:* Real food: peanut butter, cream cheese, pretzels, popcorn, almonds

9.   Healthy Portions with MyPlate

MATERIALS AND PREPARATION

Activity-Specific Materials and Preparation

Activity 9.1A

Materials

Appendix Materials

- Printed MyPlate, one for each student (Appendix D)

Additional Materials

- Large (at least 27" x 39") poster representation of MyPlate
- Real food: frozen pre-cooked meatballs (1 oz each), cooked brown rice, applesauce, broccoli, skim milk
- Large serving spoons or forks for each food item
- One plate and cup per student

Preparation

1. Cut out the plate portion of the MyPlate graphic, laminate it, and place it on each student's plate.

Activity 9.1B

Materials

Appendix Materials – None

Additional Materials

- Large (at least 27" x 39") poster representation of MyPlate
- Real food: frozen, pre-cooked, 1-oz meatballs (or food models if real food is unavailable), cooked brown rice, applesauce, broccoli, skim milk
- Large serving spoons or forks for each food item
- One plate per student with various incorrect portions, such as double protein or grains, not enough vegetables, a small glass of milk, etc.
- Tips:
  - This activity can be very fun if you add mock lab coats and scientist gloves.
  - Make the portioning of the food realistic, as student will often encounter incorrect portions in restaurants.

SECTION 9.1: HEALTHY EATING

This section focuses on the importance of eating a healthy serving of each food group at a meal. The purpose of this exercise is to get students talking about what portions and serving size mean. The lecture is very short, as much of the focus should be on actually measuring and portioning out food.

Key Points:

- Eating healthy portions means choosing the right amount of food to eat at one time to keep you healthy.
- We know we're eating healthy portions when they fit into the different sections on MyPlate. Fill half your plate with fruits and vegetables, then one quarter with protein and the other quarter with grains.

LESSON TIPS

✓ When introducing new terms, hold up corresponding flashcards.

✓ Use food pictures and models for students to reference.

1. Post the large MyPlate.gov poster at the front of the room to reference. Attach pictures of the corresponding food group onto the poster as each food group is discussed.
2. Ask the students, "Has anybody heard people talking about healthy serving sizes, or **healthy portions** (hold up flashcard)? What does that mean?"
3. Explain that eating healthy portions means choosing the right amount of food to eat at one time to keep you healthy and to keep from over-eating. It is how much of each food group your body needs at one meal.
4. Ask the students why we should choose healthy portions, because it's important not to eat too much or too little food.
5. Next, ask the students, "How do we know we're eating healthy portions?"
6. Ask the students if they remember MyPlate and explain that we can use it to plan out portion sizes, because we'll know that we're eating healthy portions when they fit into the different sections on MyPlate.
7. Show them that this means you should fill half your plate with fruits and vegetables, then one half of the other side with protein, and the other half with grains. (Refer to the MyPlate poster itself to show them each section.)

At this point in the lesson, transition into the activity.

9. Healthy Portions with MyPlate

ACTIVITY 9.1A: LEVEL 1, SKILL-BASED ACTIVITY:

In this activity, students practice filling their healthy plate using MyPlate.gov portions.

1. Set out food in large containers on an easily accessible table.
2. Distribute plates with the MyPlate graphic attached and cups to students.
3. Have students identify the food groups displayed on the table.
4. Students will then use the MyPlate portions to fill their plate and cup with the correct amount of each food group using the MyPlate graphic as a guide.
5. Have students show you which foods they chose, what group each belongs to, and where each fits on the plate.
6. Correct incorrect portions by physically adding or removing food from the plate.
7. *For an added challenge:* Once students master this with MyPlate graphics attached, take off the laminated MyPlate graphic and have them try portioning out food using a blank plate.

ACTIVITY TIPS

✓Have a correct plate ready at the front to reference.

✓You can also use other small pre-portioned meat products such as chicken tenders or fish sticks.

✓Ask additional teachers or aides to help each student measure the right amount.

✓If possible, have students go one at a time so you can coach them on accurate measurement.

✓Remind students not to eat the food!

ACTIVITY 9.1B: LEVEL 1, KNOWLEDGE-BASED ACTIVITY: "FOOD SCIENTIST"

Students will attempt to determine what is wrong with incorrectly pre-portioned plates and correct them to make a healthy plate with appropriate portion sizes.

1. Set out extra food in large containers on an easily accessible table.
2. Give each student a plate of food with incorrect portion sizes.
3. Tell student that today they will be food scientists and use what they've learned so far to determine which food portions are too small, which are too big, and which are just right.
4. Starting with one food group at a time, have students determine if the amount is correct simply by looking at the plate. If correct, they will leave it on the plate. If there's too much of something, have students move it from their plates into the large container of food at the front. If there's too little of something, have students add the food until they have the correct amount on their plates.
5. *For an added challenge:* You can use larger pieces of meat, like an 8 oz. burger or steak, so that it doesn't fit in the proportions on the plate. This will have to be cut in half and/or shared between student plates to make it the right serving size.

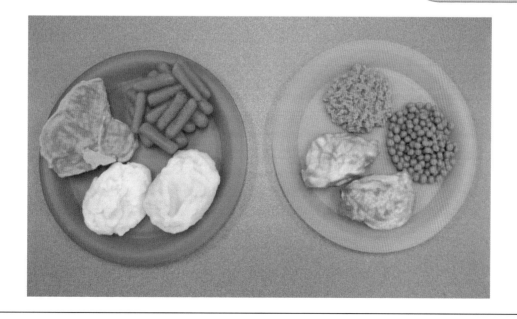

SECTION 9.2: MEASURING SNACKS AND CONDIMENTS (optional)

This section introduces additional ways that students can measure correct portions by using everyday items as guides (e.g., palm of hand, deck of cards, tennis ball).

1. Explain to the students that, for many food items that we eat as snacks, on salads, or as spreads, we have easy ways to determine what is the right amount for us to eat.
2. Here are some ways we do this:
   a. Pour nuts (almonds, peanuts) into your hand and close your fist. What fits inside is one serving of nuts.
   b. One open palm-full is one serving of pretzels.
   c. Two open palm-fulls is one serving of popcorn!
   d. A ping-pong ball is the size of one serving of peanut butter.

LESSON TIP

✓Be careful of nut allergies!

"KEEP MOVING"

Take 15 minutes at the end of class to participate in an interactive physical activity (see Appendix F for ideas).

PHYSICAL ACTIVITY TIP
Reinforce how physical activity goes hand-in-hand with good nutrition for health.

If resources are available, try to conclude each lesson with a taste test. Taste test ideas:

· **Sampler of (small) servings from each of the five food groups, fit into a small pre-portioned plate**

TASTE TEST TIP
Reinforce the importance of portion size in the taste test.

DAILY WRAP-UP (Appendix E)

Eat a new food from one of the food groups.

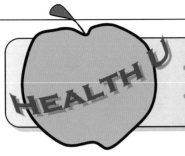

10   Eating Out & Around Town

OVERVIEW

The goal of this lesson is to use knowledge from lessons 1-9 to choose the healthiest foods at a restaurant. Students will discuss eating at a restaurant, then utilize role play and audience participation in a skit about a parent and child eating out together. You will need at least 3 adults (non-students) for this exercise and will use the classroom as the stage for the skit.

LEARNING OBJECTIVES

At the end of the session, students will be able to:
- ✓ Explain how to identify the healthy food options on a restaurant menu
- ✓ Apply previous knowledge from lessons 1-9 while eating in a restaurant (including healthy drinks, main dishes, and sides)

MATERIALS AND PREPARATION

General Materials for the Lesson
Appendix Materials
- Pictures of salads with dressing on it and with dressing on the side (Appendix C)
- "Take Home Ideas" worksheet (Appendix E)
- Physical activity ideas (Appendix F)

Additional Materials (see Guidelines for Use, p. iii, for tips on obtaining these)
- "To go" container(s) from a local restaurant (for leftovers)

10. Eating Out & Around Town

MATERIALS AND PREPARATION

Activity-Specific Materials and Preparation
Activity 10.1
Materials
Appendix Materials
- Sulley's menu cover (Appendix P)
- Restaurant skit script, 1 per actor (Appendix Q)

Additional Materials
- Food item props "ordered" by the actors (use food models): 3 pieces grilled chicken, grilled fish, 3 sides of dressing, 1 order French fries, broccoli, 2 salads
- Non-food props: bread basket, notepad and pen, tray, 3 plates and 2 cups, to-go container, tablecloth, napkins, utensils
- 2 folders with Sulley's menu covers taped to front

Preparation
- Use the front of the classroom as a stage with:
    - Stage Left: 2 chairs side-by-side, facing crowd (these will be the seats in the "car")
    - Stage Right:
        - Small table set for dinner for 2
        - Easel and white board with specials written on it: Fried chicken with French fries and coleslaw, Grilled ginger soy salmon
- Have a staging area in the back or outside of the classroom for the remaining props

SECTION 10.1: CHOOSING HEALTHY OPTIONS AT A RESTAURANT

In this section, you will discuss how to make healthy choices at a restaurant.

Key Points:
- Making healthy choices at a restaurant can be hard, because most restaurants often prepare the food with lots of extra sugar and fat, serve foods that aren't healthy choices, and/or give you way too much food.
- However, there are some strategies you can use to help you make healthier choices at restaurants.

1. Start by asking students, "Who likes to eat at restaurants? What are some of your favorite restaurants?"
2. Then ask, "Is it ever hard to find healthy options when eating at a restaurant?" Explain that it can be hard to make healthy choices at restaurants because they often prepare the food with lots of extra sugar and fat and serve foods that aren't healthy choices. Also, they usually give you lots of food (the portions are really big).
3. Ask the students if they can think of ways they could make healthier choices at a restaurant.
4. Discuss each of the following tips (which can be written on the board for reference):
   a. Read the menu before going to the restaurant to find the healthiest choices.
   b. Choose grilled, baked, or steamed options.
   c. Choose vegetables or fruit as a side dish.
   d. Ask for the sauce (mayo, dressing) on the side. Review the pictures of the salad with dressing and the salad with dressing on the side (Appendix C).
   e. Choose water, seltzer, unsweetened tea, or low-fat milk. Those free refills of soda can really add up!
   f. Split a meal with someone, or take half of it home in a doggie bag. Many restaurants give you way too much food!
   g. Desserts and appetizers are fun, but think of them like treats! Enjoy them only once in a while.

At this point in the lesson, transition into the activity.

LESSON TIPS

✓ To encourage participation, have each student identify a restaurant they like.

✓ Show the students an example of a container that restaurants use for leftovers.

✓ Depending on the instructor's preference, the discussion can happen during or after the skit.

ACTIVITY 10.1A: LEVEL 1, KNOWLEDGE-CENTERED ACTIVITY:

In this activity, students watch a skit (Appendix Q) and help the "actors" make healthy choices at a fictional restaurant.

Note: You will need at least 3 adults (non-students) for this exercise. The "Commentator" and "Waitress" can be played by the same person, or you can have a fourth person participate.

1. Introduce the actors and skit to the class.
2. Start the skit.

ACTIVITY TIPS

✓ Be sure you have enough staff to be the actors in the skit.

✓ Practice the skit ahead of time.

✓ Encourage audience participation to make it fun! For example, stop the skit and ask for suggestions.

✓ After running through the skit, if time permits, have students make up their own skit. This can be very enlightening because you see what messages they have taken away from the lessons.

"KEEP MOVING"

Take 15 minutes at the end of class to participate in an interactive physical activity (see Appendix F for ideas).

PHYSICAL ACTIVITY TIP
Ask students what physical activities they've done and whether they've noticed anything positive when doing physical activity.

If resources are available, try to conclude each lesson with a taste test. Taste test ideas:

· **Healthy to-go item(s) from a restaurant or fast food place**

TASTE TEST TIP
Choose a restaurant where the students like to eat and find a healthy option from the menu.

DAILY WRAP-UP (Appendix E)

Find a healthy item at your favorite restaurant.

APPENDIX INSTRUCTIONS

The appendix is available in the form of downloadable/printable PDFs that can be accessed via password at the following website:

Website: http://healthu.neindex.org

Username: healthu

Password: !Appendix13

For any technical problems, please contact the first author at linda.bandini@umassmed.edu.

Appendix Summary

Appendix A: Flashcards. This section contains flashcards of all of the vocabulary words used in the lessons.

Appendix B: Food Group Cards. This section contains 5 large cards, one for each food group, with pictures of items within that food group.

Appendix C: Pictures. This section contains pictures of a number of different foods used in various lessons.

Appendix D: MyPlate. This section contains a sample graphic from the ChooseMyPlate.gov website used in various lessons.

Appendix E: Take Home Ideas. This section contains a worksheet for students to take home that highlights what they learned about healthy eating, what foods they tried in class, as well as foods they will try at home. This is used at the end of each lesson.

Appendix F: Physical Activity Ideas. This section contains a short list of physical activities to get students moving.

Appendix G: Eat a Rainbow Placemat. This section contains a placemat that has a plate with the grain group and meat and beans group already filled used in Lesson 2.

Appendix H: Sample Menu. This section contains a sample menu for students to practice picking out healthy items at a restaurant used in Lesson 2.

Appendix I: Whole Grain Model. This section contains a visual of the three parts of a whole grain used in Lesson 3.

Appendix J: BINGO supplies. This section contains seven different BINGO boards, five cards with different protein categories, and a card for each BINGO letter used in Lesson 3.

Appendix K: 3 Sample Plates. This section contains three plates representing three different meals: chicken; chicken and rice; chicken, rice, and vegetables. These are used in Lesson 4.

Appendix L: Mixed Dish Examples. This section contains the parts to three different mixed dishes: pizza, a sandwich, and pasta. These are used in Lesson 4.

Appendix M: "Switch-A-Roo" Materials. This section contains pictures of unhealthy and healthy foods that make up the four different meals of the "Switch-A-Roo" game and a "Switch-A-Roo Ideas" handout for students to take home to their parents. These are used in Lesson 7.

Appendix N: "Go Snack" Cards. This section contains 63 cards: 27 pairs of healthy snack cards and 9 single unhealthy snack cards used in Lesson 8.

Appendix O: Jersey and Score Boards. This section contains a jersey, a scoreboard, and sample snack cards for students to take home and bring back to report their snacks. These are used in Lesson 8.

Appendix P: Sulley's Menu Cover. This section contains a menu cover for the restaurant used in the skit in Lesson 10.

Appendix Q: Restaurant Skit Script. This section contains the script used for the restaurant skit in Lesson 10.

Appendix R: Photo Sources. This section contains the sources for all of the photos used in the curriculum.